MYSTIC
WELLNESS LAB

ELEVATING WELLNESS THROUGH SCIENCE & MYSTICISM

THE MYSTIC THERAPY GUIDEBOOK – UNLOCKING THE SECRETS OF SELF-HEALING

MYSTIC WELLNESS LAB

THE MYSTIC THERAPY GUIDEBOOK – UNLOCKING THE SECRETS OF SELF-HEALING

A JOURNEY INTO ANCIENT WISDOM, ENERGY HEALING, AND CONSCIOUS TRANSFORMATION

Embarking on a journey into ancient wisdom, energy healing, and conscious transformation is akin to stepping into a vibrant tapestry woven with the threads of history, spirituality, and personal empowerment. Throughout the ages, countless cultures have recognized the profound interconnectedness of mind, body, and spirit. These teachings have been passed down through generations, offering us a treasure trove of insights that can illuminate our path to self-healing. As we delve into this rich reservoir of knowledge, we unlock the secrets that empower us to reclaim our innate ability to heal and transform.

Energy healing practices, deeply rooted in ancient traditions, serve as powerful catalysts for personal growth and transformation. From the gentle flow of Reiki to the dynamic movements of Tai Chi, these modalities harness the life force energy that permeates all living beings. By learning to channel and balance this energy, we can release blockages, harmonize our emotions, and rejuvenate our physical bodies.

This journey becomes an intimate dance with our inner selves, as we cultivate awareness and learn to listen to the subtle messages our bodies convey. Embracing energy healing not only enhances our well-being but also fosters a deeper connection to the universal energies that surround us.

As we explore the concept of conscious transformation, we begin to understand the profound impact of our thoughts, beliefs, and intentions on our healing journey. Ancient wisdom teaches us that we are not merely passive recipients of life's experiences; rather, we are active co-creators of our reality. By harnessing the power of mindfulness and intention, we can reshape our narratives, shedding limiting beliefs and embracing a more expansive view of ourselves. This conscious shift opens the door to new possibilities, inviting us to step boldly into our authentic selves and realize our fullest potential.

Integrating ancient wisdom into our modern lives requires a commitment to self-discovery and a willingness to embrace change. This journey is not always easy; it demands courage and vulnerability as we confront the shadows of our past and the fears that may hold us back. However, each step taken toward healing is a step toward liberation. With every practice, whether it's meditation, breathwork, or energy alignment, we cultivate a deeper understanding of ourselves and the world around us. In this sacred space, we learn to honor our own journeys while supporting one another in the collective quest for healing and transformation.

Ultimately, the journey into ancient wisdom, energy healing, and conscious transformation is a celebration of life itself. It invites us to awaken to the beauty of our existence and embrace the myriad ways in which we can heal ourselves and each other. As we unlock the secrets of self-healing, we become beacons of light in a world that often feels shrouded in darkness. Together, we embark on this extraordinary adventure, harnessing the gifts of the past to forge a brighter, more harmonious future. Let us step boldly into our power and embrace the divine potential that resides within us all.

CHAPTER 1: THE MYSTICAL PATH TO SELF-HEALING

* * *

What is Mystic Therapy? The Fusion of Ancient Wisdom and Modern Science

Mystic therapy emerges as a captivating blend of ancient wisdom and contemporary scientific understanding, creating a holistic approach to self-healing that resonates with the needs of today's seekers. Drawing from centuries-old practices like meditation, energy healing, and herbal medicine, mystic therapy revitalizes these age-old techniques through the lens of modern psychology and neuroscience. This fusion not only validates the effectiveness of traditional methods but also provides a deeper understanding of how these practices influence our minds and bodies, making it an exciting field for anyone on a journey of self-discovery and healing.

At its core, mystic therapy recognizes that we are more than just our physical bodies; we are intricate webs of energy, emotion, and spirit. By engaging with ancient philosophies, such as those found in Eastern traditions, mystic therapy encourages individuals to explore their inner landscapes and connect with their true selves. This exploration often leads to profound insights and transformative healing experiences. The integration of modern science allows us to appreciate the physiological benefits of these practices, such as reduced stress, improved mental clarity, and enhanced emotional resilience, thus appealing to both the heart and the mind.

Practitioners of mystic therapy utilize a variety of techniques tailored to individual needs, including guided imagery, sound healing, and breathwork. Each method serves as a bridge between the physical and spiritual realms, inviting practitioners to deepen their self-awareness and foster a sense of inner peace. For example, sound healing employs frequencies that resonate with our body's natural rhythms, promoting relaxation and healing. This innovative approach highlights the power of intention and the potential for self-healing that lies within each of us, inspiring individuals to take an active role in their wellness.

Moreover, mystic therapy emphasizes the interconnectedness of all aspects of life—mind, body, spirit, and environment. By acknowledging this profound connection, individuals are encouraged to cultivate a holistic lifestyle that nurtures their overall well-being. This can include mindful eating, connecting with nature, and fostering positive relationships. The modern scientific research supporting these practices enhances their credibility, making mystic therapy an increasingly popular choice for those seeking sustainable healing methods that align with their values and beliefs.

In conclusion, mystic therapy stands as a testament to the timeless quest for healing and understanding that transcends generations. By harmonizing ancient wisdom with modern scientific insights, this approach opens the door to a transformative journey of self-healing that resonates deeply with those who seek to unlock their potential. As more individuals turn to mystic therapy, they find not only relief from their ailments but also a path toward greater self-awareness, empowerment, and connection to the universe at large. Embrace this synergy of knowledge and experience the incredible possibilities that await on your journey of self-discovery and healing.

Understanding the Body's Natural Ability to Heal

* * *

The human body possesses an incredible innate ability to heal itself, a phenomenon that has fascinated scientists, healers, and the spiritually inclined for centuries. This miraculous capacity for self-repair is rooted in our biology, where complex systems work in harmony to restore balance, fight infections, and mend injuries. Understanding this natural ability can empower individuals to tap into their own healing potential, fostering a deeper connection between mind, body, and spirit. By recognizing the body as a dynamic, self-sustaining organism, we begin to appreciate the profound wisdom it holds.

At the core of this healing power lies the immune system, a sophisticated network of cells, tissues, and organs that defend the body against harmful invaders. This system operates tirelessly, responding to threats with remarkable precision. When you cut your finger, for instance, a cascade of biochemical signals is initiated, summoning white blood cells to the site of injury, where they work diligently to prevent infection and promote healing. By acknowledging the efficiency of this process, we can cultivate a sense of trust in our bodies, reinforcing the belief that healing is not only possible but is a natural state of being.

Beyond the physical mechanisms, the mind plays a crucial role in the healing journey. Our thoughts, emotions, and beliefs can either support or hinder our body's natural processes. The practice of mindfulness, meditation, and positive affirmations can significantly enhance the body's ability to heal. By fostering a positive mindset and reducing stress, we create an internal environment conducive to recovery. This interplay between the mental and physical realms highlights the importance of holistic approaches that honor the interconnectedness of our experiences.

Moreover, lifestyle choices can profoundly impact our body's healing capabilities. Nutrition, exercise, and sleep are foundational elements that either nourish or deplete our systems. A diet rich in whole foods, full of antioxidants and essential nutrients, provides the building blocks necessary for repair and regeneration. Regular physical activity not only strengthens the body but also boosts mood and mental clarity, while restorative sleep allows for vital processes to occur. By consciously making choices that support our health, we activate and amplify our natural healing mechanisms.

Finally, embracing alternative therapies can further unlock the secrets of self-healing. Practices such as acupuncture, aromatherapy, and energy healing have been utilized for centuries to enhance the body's innate abilities. These modalities tap into the subtle energies that flow through us, facilitating balance and harmony. By exploring and integrating these diverse healing practices, we expand our toolkit and invite a richer, more vibrant experience of health. Understanding the body's natural ability to heal is not merely an intellectual exercise; it is an invitation to embark on a transformative journey toward self-discovery and empowerment.

How Energy, Mindset, and Lifestyle Shape Well-Being

* * *

Energy, mindset, and lifestyle are the foundational pillars of well-being, each intricately woven into the fabric of our daily lives. Energy, in its many forms, is the life force that propels us forward, influencing our physical health, emotional state, and spiritual connection. When we harness positive energy, we create a vibrant atmosphere that nurtures our growth and healing. By cultivating an environment filled with love, gratitude, and positivity, we allow our energy to flourish, enabling us to tap into our fullest potential.

Mindset serves as the lens through which we perceive the world and our place within it. A growth-oriented mindset empowers us to embrace challenges and view setbacks as opportunities for learning and transformation. This shift in perspective is crucial for personal development and self-healing. By fostering an optimistic outlook, we can reshape our beliefs, releasing limiting thoughts that inhibit our progress. An empowered mindset not only enhances our resilience but also attracts positive experiences, reinforcing our journey toward well-being.

Lifestyle choices play an equally significant role in shaping our well-being. Every decision, from the foods we consume to the activities we engage in, impacts our physical and mental health. Adopting a balanced lifestyle that prioritizes nutrition, exercise, and mindfulness is essential for maintaining harmony within ourselves. Simple practices like daily movement, nourishing meals, and moments of stillness can significantly elevate our overall well-being. By consciously choosing habits that support our health, we create a sustainable path to self-healing.

The interplay of energy, mindset, and lifestyle creates a powerful synergy that enhances our well-being. When we align our thoughts with positive energy and support them with healthy choices, we unlock the potential for profound transformation. This holistic approach to self-healing allows us to connect deeply with ourselves, fostering a sense of inner peace and fulfillment. By recognizing the interconnectedness of these elements, we cultivate a life imbued with purpose and joy.

As we embark on the journey of self-healing, let us embrace the dynamic relationship between energy, mindset, and lifestyle. Each step we take toward nurturing these aspects brings us closer to achieving harmony and balance in our lives. By staying attuned to our energy, maintaining a positive mindset, and making conscious lifestyle choices, we empower ourselves to thrive. Together, let us unlock the secrets of well-being and step into a brighter, more vibrant existence.

CHAPTER 2: THE HUMAN ENERGY SYSTEM – UNLOCKING THE POWER WITHIN

* * *

The Subtle Energy Body: Chakras, Meridians, and the Aura

The subtle energy body is a fascinating aspect of our being, intricately woven into the fabric of our existence. It includes the chakras, meridians, and the aura, forming an energetic network that influences our physical, emotional, and spiritual well-being. Understanding this energy body is essential for anyone looking to unlock the secrets of self-healing. By tapping into these subtle energies, we can harmonize our inner selves and cultivate a life filled with vitality and purpose.

Chakras are the vital energy centers located along the spine, each corresponding to different aspects of our lives. There are seven main chakras, each with its unique vibrational frequency and function. The root chakra connects us to the earth, grounding us in stability, while the crown chakra links us to higher consciousness and spiritual enlightenment. By learning to balance these energy centers, we can release blockages that hinder our growth, allowing us to thrive emotionally and spiritually. Embracing practices such as meditation, yoga, and breathwork can help activate and align these chakras, enhancing our overall health and vitality.

Meridians, the pathways through which life energy, or Qi, flows, play a crucial role in maintaining our energetic balance. Originating from traditional Chinese medicine, these channels connect the internal organs and systems, facilitating the smooth flow of energy throughout the body. When the meridians are clear, energy flows freely, promoting optimal health and well-being. However, stress, trauma, and unhealthy habits can lead to blockages. Techniques such as acupuncture, acupressure, and energy healing can help clear these pathways, restoring balance and harmony to our subtle energy body.

The aura, a luminous field surrounding our physical body, reflects our emotional state and overall health. This energy field is a vibrant tapestry of colors and vibrations that communicates our thoughts, feelings, and spiritual condition to the world around us. By becoming more aware of our aura, we can gain insights into our mental and emotional patterns, as well as those of others. Practices such as energy cleansing, visualization, and mindful awareness can help us maintain a vibrant and healthy aura, fostering a greater connection to ourselves and the universe.

Incorporating the understanding of the subtle energy body into our daily lives can lead to profound transformations. By nurturing our chakras, meridians, and aura, we open ourselves to a deeper level of self-awareness and healing. This journey is not just about physical health; it's about embracing the interconnectedness of mind, body, and spirit. With curiosity and enthusiasm, we can explore these energy systems and unlock the secrets they hold, empowering ourselves on the path to self-healing and holistic well-being.

The Science of Biofields and Electromagnetic Energy

* * *

The exploration of biofields and electromagnetic energy opens a fascinating portal into the unseen forces that influence our well-being. Biofields refer to the energetic fields surrounding and permeating living beings, acting as a bridge between the physical and the energetic realms. These fields are not merely abstract concepts; they can be measured and studied scientifically, shedding light on how our bodies interact with the energy around us. As we delve into this captivating subject, we uncover the profound ways in which our biofields impact our health, emotions, and spiritual vitality.

At the core of this science lies the understanding that everything in the universe, including our bodies, vibrates at specific frequencies. This electromagnetic energy is a fundamental aspect of our existence, and it plays a crucial role in regulating our biological functions. Research in fields such as quantum physics and bioenergetics reveals that our cells communicate through these electromagnetic signals, influencing everything from cellular health to emotional states. When our biofields are in harmony, we experience balance and wellness; however, disruptions can lead to various ailments, both physical and psychological.

One of the most exciting aspects of biofields is their responsiveness to intention and consciousness. Studies have shown that our thoughts and emotions can significantly alter the energy patterns within our biofields. For instance, positive intentions can enhance our vibrational frequencies, promoting healing and vitality. Conversely, negative emotions can create blockages and distortions that may manifest as physical symptoms. This interplay between consciousness and electromagnetic energy highlights the power we hold in our self-healing journeys, inviting us to harness our inner potential.

Healing modalities such as Reiki, acupuncture, and therapeutic touch are grounded in the principles of biofields and electromagnetic energy. These practices aim to restore balance to the biofield, facilitating the flow of energy throughout the body. Practitioners often report remarkable transformations in their clients as they release stagnant energy and encourage a harmonious exchange of electromagnetic signals. This ancient wisdom, now supported by modern scientific research, empowers us to embrace healing practices that align with our energetic nature.

As we continue to unlock the secrets of self-healing, understanding the science of biofields and electromagnetic energy becomes essential. By recognizing the interconnectedness of our physical, emotional, and energetic selves, we can cultivate a holistic approach to health and well-being. Embracing this knowledge not only enhances our healing practices but also deepens our connection to the vibrant energy that surrounds us. As we embark on this journey, we are reminded that we are not merely passive recipients of energy; we are active participants in the dance of life, capable of influencing our biofields and, ultimately, our destinies.

How to Strengthen and Balance Your Energy Field

* * *

Strengthening and balancing your energy field is a transformative journey that can elevate your overall well-being and empower your self-healing abilities. To embark on this adventure, begin by cultivating awareness of your energy body. This involves tuning into your feelings, thoughts, and physical sensations. Spend a few moments each day in quiet reflection, focusing on your breath and observing the subtle shifts within you. As you become more attuned to your energy, you'll notice areas that feel dense or stagnant, indicating where you may need to direct your attention and intention.

One of the most effective practices for enhancing your

energy field is through grounding. Grounding connects you to the Earth's energy, providing stability and nourishment. Simple activities such as walking barefoot on grass, hugging a tree, or meditating outdoors can help you establish this vital connection. Visualize roots extending from your feet into the Earth, drawing up pure, revitalizing energy. As you ground yourself, focus on releasing any negativity or stress, allowing it to dissolve into the Earth, which transforms it into positive energy.

Incorporating energy-clearing techniques into your routine is essential for maintaining a balanced energy field. Techniques such as smudging with sage, using crystals, or practicing sound healing can help clear any stagnant or negative energy. Each method has its unique benefits, so explore various options to find what resonates with you. For instance, placing crystals like amethyst or clear quartz in your living space can create a harmonious environment, while the sound of a singing bowl can uplift and cleanse your energy. Make these practices a regular part of your self-care ritual.

Another powerful way to strengthen your energy field is through the practice of visualization. Visualization involves creating vivid mental images to manifest desired outcomes or to reinforce your energetic boundaries. Imagine a protective bubble of light surrounding you, shimmering with vibrant colors. This bubble not only deflects negativity but also amplifies your energy, helping you feel more confident and centered. Regularly visualizing this protective shield can enhance your resilience against external influences, allowing you to maintain your balance amidst life's challenges.

Lastly, nurturing your body through mindful nutrition and movement is crucial for a vibrant energy field. Eating a balanced diet rich in whole foods, staying hydrated, and engaging in regular physical activity can significantly impact your energy levels. Consider incorporating practices like yoga or tai chi, which not only promote physical health but also align your energy centers. As you strengthen your physical body, your energy field naturally follows suit, creating a harmonious balance that supports your self-healing journey. Embrace these practices with enthusiasm, and watch as your energy field flourishes, leading you toward a more empowered and vibrant existence.

CHAPTER 3: BREATHWORK AS A GATEWAY TO HEALING

* * *

The Power of Pranayama and Conscious Breathing

Pranayama and conscious breathing are transformative practices that hold the potential to unlock deep states of healing and self-awareness. As we navigate through the stresses of modern life, the power of our breath often goes unnoticed, yet it serves as a bridge connecting our physical body, mind, and spirit. By harnessing the techniques of pranayama, we can tap into an ancient wisdom that invites peace, clarity, and vitality into our daily existence. This subchapter invites you to explore the profound impact that intentional breathing can have on your overall well-being.

At the core of pranayama lies the understanding that breath is life. Each inhalation brings in fresh energy, while each exhalation allows us to release what no longer serves us. This dynamic exchange not only nourishes our body with oxygen but also purifies our emotional and mental states. As we cultivate conscious breathing practices, we learn to regulate our autonomic nervous system, reducing stress and anxiety while promoting relaxation and mindfulness. Imagine the freedom that comes from mastering your breath

—a tool that is always available to you, ready to ground you in moments of chaos.

Engaging with pranayama can lead to heightened self-awareness and a deeper connection to our inner selves. Through various techniques such as Nadi Shodhana (alternate nostril breathing) or Ujjayi (victorious breath), practitioners can experience shifts in energy and consciousness. These methods are not just about inhaling and exhaling; they are gateways to exploring the very essence of our being. As we practice, we may uncover the layers of tension and emotional blockages that reside within, allowing us to release and heal through the power of breath. This journey into self-discovery is exhilarating, as every breath becomes an opportunity to connect with our true nature.

Moreover, pranayama can greatly enhance our physical health. Scientific studies have shown that conscious breathing can improve lung function, increase oxygenation of the blood, and even lower blood pressure. By integrating these practices into our daily routines, we equip ourselves with tools to combat fatigue and enhance vitality. Feel the invigorating energy that arises from deep, intentional breaths, and let it serve as a reminder that our breath is a potent source of life force. The practice of pranayama is not merely an exercise; it is a healing modality that empowers us to reclaim our health and vitality.

As you delve into the world of pranayama and conscious breathing, remember that consistency is key. Start with a few minutes each day, gradually increasing the duration and complexity of your practice as you become more comfortable. Embrace the journey with enthusiasm and curiosity, for every breath taken with intention can lead to profound insights and transformation. This powerful practice invites you to witness the magic that unfolds when you consciously engage with your breath, turning simple inhalations and exhalations into a sacred ritual of self-healing. The power to heal, rejuvenate, and thrive lies within you—waiting to be awakened through the art of pranayama.

How Oxygenation Enhances Mental and Physical Health

* * *

Oxygenation plays a pivotal role in enhancing both mental and physical health, acting as a vital fuel for our bodies and minds. The moment we inhale, oxygen enters our bloodstream, delivering life-sustaining energy to every cell. This process invigorates not just our physical health but also clears our mental pathways, allowing for sharper focus and heightened creativity. Imagine feeling a surge of vitality coursing through you; that's the magic of oxygenation, transforming fatigue into exuberance and promoting a sense of well-being that resonates deeply within.

When we think about mental clarity, oxygenation is an often-overlooked component. Our brains, which consume about 20% of the oxygen we breathe, thrive on this essential element. Enhanced oxygen levels improve cognitive functions, enabling us to process information more efficiently and make decisions with confidence. This boost in mental agility can be especially beneficial during stressful situations, where clarity of thought is paramount. By simply focusing on our breath and consciously taking in more oxygen, we can pave the way for a more resilient mind, ready to tackle challenges with enthusiasm.

Physical health, too, experiences a tremendous uplift through optimized oxygenation. Oxygen is crucial for cellular respiration, the process by which our bodies convert nutrients into energy. This energy not only fuels our daily activities but is essential for muscle recovery and overall physical endurance. Engaging in activities that promote oxygen flow, such as exercise, yoga, or even mindful breathing, can lead to improved cardiovascular health and increased stamina. The exhilaration that accompanies physical activity is closely tied to our oxygen levels, illustrating the profound connection between breath and vitality.

Moreover, the benefits of proper oxygenation extend to emotional health, creating a harmonious balance within. When we breathe deeply and effectively, we stimulate the production of endorphins, often referred to as the "feel-good" hormones. This process not only elevates our mood but also helps alleviate symptoms of anxiety and depression. By incorporating breathwork into our daily routines, we can cultivate a sense of inner peace, allowing our emotional landscape to flourish. The simple act of focusing on our breath can become a powerful tool for transforming our emotional states and enhancing our overall quality of life.

In conclusion, oxygenation is a fundamental aspect of our well-being, intricately linked to our mental, physical, and emotional health. By recognizing its importance and actively engaging in practices that enhance oxygen flow, we unlock the door to a more vibrant existence. Whether through mindful breathing, physical activity, or holistic therapies, embracing oxygenation can lead us on a transformative journey toward self-healing. The energy and clarity that come from fully utilizing our breath are not just beneficial—they are the keys to living our most radiant lives.

Simple Breathwork Practices for Energy and Calmness

* * *

Breathwork is a powerful yet often overlooked tool in our journey toward self-healing. By simply engaging in conscious breathing, we can harness energy and cultivate a profound sense of calmness. These simple practices can be easily integrated into your daily routine, allowing you to tap into your inner vitality while simultaneously soothing your mind and spirit. The beauty of breathwork lies in its accessibility; anyone, regardless of experience or background, can utilize these techniques to enhance their well-being.

One of the easiest methods to start your breathwork practice is through deep abdominal breathing, also known as diaphragmatic breathing. Find a comfortable position, either seated or lying down, and place one hand on your belly. Inhale deeply through your nose, allowing your abdomen to rise as you fill your lungs with air. Hold that breath for a moment, and then exhale slowly through your mouth, feeling your belly fall. Repeat this cycle for several minutes, focusing on the rise and fall of your abdomen. Not only does this technique energize your body, but it also activates the parasympathetic nervous system, promoting relaxation and reducing stress.

Another invigorating practice to explore is the 4-7-8 breathing technique. This simple yet effective method can quickly shift your mental state and invigorate your spirit. To practice, inhale quietly through your nose for a count of four, hold your breath for a count of seven, and then exhale completely through your mouth for a count of eight. This rhythmic pattern of breathing can be repeated four times in succession. As you engage in this practice, visualize each breath filling you with energy and each exhale releasing tension and negativity. This technique not only boosts your energy levels but also calms the mind, making it an excellent tool for those moments when life feels overwhelming.

For those seeking a more meditative approach, consider practicing box breathing. This technique encourages mindfulness while stimulating both energy and tranquility. Imagine a square as you breathe: inhale for a count of four, hold that breath for four, exhale for four, and then pause for another count of four before inhaling again. Visualizing the square can help center your thoughts and bring clarity to your day. Each breath becomes a step toward balance, allowing you to cultivate a sense of stability amidst the chaos of everyday life.

Lastly, the practice of alternate nostril breathing, or Nadi Shodhana, is an incredible way to harmonize the body's energy channels. Sit comfortably and use your right thumb to close your right nostril. Inhale deeply through the left nostril, then close the left nostril with your right ring finger, releasing the right nostril to exhale through it. Inhale through the right nostril, close it, and exhale through the left. This cycle can be repeated for several minutes. This practice not only energizes your body but also calms the mind, creating a harmonious balance within yourself.

Incorporating these simple breathwork practices into your daily routine can be transformative. Whether you seek energy, calmness, or clarity, the breath is your ally. Embrace these techniques with enthusiasm and curiosity, and watch how they enhance your journey toward self-healing. Your breath is a bridge to a more vibrant and peaceful existence, guiding you toward the profound wisdom that lies within.

CHAPTER 4: THE HEALING POWER OF WATER AND HYDRATION

* * *

How Water Affects Energy, Consciousness, and Cellular Health

Water is often referred to as the essence of life, and its impact on our energy, consciousness, and cellular health cannot be overstated. Every drop we consume is a vital component that fuels our bodies, influences our mental clarity, and enhances our overall well-being. When we hydrate adequately, we experience a surge of energy that can propel us through our daily tasks, invigorate our spirits, and elevate our moods. This dynamic relationship between water and energy is crucial for anyone seeking to maximize their potential and embrace a life filled with vitality.

The connection between water and consciousness is equally fascinating. Water is known to be an excellent conductor of energy, facilitating communication within our cells and between our mind and body. As we drink water, it not only hydrates us but also clears mental fog and sharpens our focus. Many spiritual traditions recognize the importance of water in meditation and mindfulness practices, where it serves as a conduit for accessing higher states of awareness. When we are adequately hydrated, we are better equipped to tap into our intuition and foster a deeper connection with our inner selves.

Cellular health is fundamentally linked to the quality and quantity of the water we consume. Our cells require water to function optimally, as it plays a crucial role in nutrient absorption, waste elimination, and maintaining structural integrity. Dehydration can lead to cellular dysfunction, resulting in fatigue, diminished cognitive performance, and a host of health issues. Conversely, when we prioritize hydration, we empower our cells to thrive, enhancing their ability to communicate and regenerate. This rejuvenation process is essential for anyone on a journey of self-healing and transformation.

Moreover, water's unique properties extend to its ability to carry and transmit energy. Each sip we take can be infused with intention and mindfulness, allowing us to harness its potential for healing. By incorporating practices such as blessing our water or visualizing healing light as we drink, we can amplify its effects on our bodies and consciousness. This practice not only enhances our hydration experience but also transforms water into a powerful ally in our quest for health and spiritual growth.

In conclusion, understanding the profound effects of water on energy, consciousness, and cellular health is a crucial step in the journey of self-healing. By embracing the transformative power of hydration, we can unlock new levels of vitality and awareness. As we nurture our bodies with pure, intentional water, we create a solid foundation for holistic wellness, allowing us to thrive in every aspect of our lives. The path to self-healing is illuminated by the simple yet profound act of honoring our relationship with water.

Structured and Energized Water for Detox and Vitality

* * *

Structured and energized water is an exciting frontier in the journey toward detoxification and vitality. This special form of water, which has been restructured at a molecular level, is believed to carry enhanced properties that can significantly boost our health and well-being. Just as nature intended, when water is treated through various methods—like vortexing, freezing, or the use of crystals—it can take on a more harmonious structure that aligns with the vibrational frequencies of life itself. Imagine drinking water that is not just a thirst quencher but a life force that invigorates your cells and enhances your overall energy.

When we consume structured and energized water, we introduce a powerful ally into our detoxification process. Traditional water can often carry impurities and imbalances, but structured water is thought to be free from these burdens, allowing your body to release toxins more efficiently. This water can help to flush out harmful substances, support kidney function, and promote better digestion. By incorporating structured water into your daily routine, you can transform your body into a more efficient detoxification system, paving the way for increased vitality and wellness.

Moreover, the benefits of energized water extend beyond detoxification. The revitalizing properties of this water can enhance hydration, leading to improved energy levels and mental clarity. Many people report feeling more alert and focused after regularly consuming structured water, as it optimizes cellular hydration and nutrient absorption. This increased energy can empower you to engage more fully with your daily activities, whether that means pursuing personal passions, enhancing your physical fitness, or deepening your spiritual practices.

In addition to its physical benefits, the act of drinking structured and energized water can be a mindful ritual that promotes emotional and spiritual well-being. As you sip this revitalizing elixir, take a moment to set intentions for your health and vitality. Visualize the water flowing through your body, cleansing and uplifting every cell. This simple practice can create a deep connection with your body's innate wisdom, reinforcing your commitment to self-care and holistic healing.

Ultimately, structured and energized water represents a remarkable tool in our quest for detoxification and vitality. By embracing this extraordinary form of water, we open ourselves up to a world of potential for healing and rejuvenation. It's a reminder that the simplest elements of nature can hold profound power when we treat them with respect and intention. Dive into the transformative effects of structured and energized water, and watch as it elevates not just your health, but your entire experience of life.

Water Rituals for Emotional and Spiritual Cleansing

* * *

Water rituals have been a cornerstone of emotional and spiritual cleansing across cultures and traditions for centuries. The fluidity and adaptability of water make it a perfect symbol for transformation and renewal. By engaging in these rituals, individuals can release pent-up emotions, clear stagnant energy, and invite a fresh wave of positivity into their lives. Whether through a simple bath, a flowing river, or a ceremonial practice, the act of immersing oneself in water can serve as a powerful catalyst for healing.

One of the most accessible forms of water ritual is the cleansing bath. By adding elements such as sea salt, essential oils, or herbal infusions, you can create a sacred space that nurtures both your body and spirit. As you soak in the warmth, visualize the water washing away your worries and negative thoughts. Each drop becomes a symbol of emotional release, helping to alleviate stress and anxiety. This ritual can be enhanced by incorporating meditation or affirmations, allowing you to deepen your connection to the water and its healing properties.

For those seeking a more communal experience, participating in a water ceremony can be profoundly transformative. These gatherings often involve group prayers, offerings, or even dances by a body of water, such as a river or lake. The collective energy of participants amplifies the intention behind the ritual, creating a powerful wave of healing that can ripple through the community. Engaging with others in this sacred practice fosters a sense of belonging and connection, reminding us that we are not alone in our journeys of emotional and spiritual cleansing.

If you live near the ocean, consider taking a moment to connect with the waves. Stand at the water's edge, breathe deeply, and allow the rhythm of the tides to synchronize with your heartbeat. As you watch the waves roll in and out, focus on the ebb and flow of your own emotions. Imagine each wave pulling away your fears and doubts, leaving you refreshed and revitalized. This simple yet profound connection with the ocean serves as a reminder of the resilience and adaptability within us all.

Incorporating water rituals into your daily life can create a sustained practice of emotional and spiritual cleansing. Whether it's sipping water mindfully, taking a shower with intention, or simply appreciating the beauty of a rain shower, these small acts can have a significant impact on your overall well-being. By honoring water as a sacred element, you invite healing into your life, allowing it to flow freely and transform your emotional landscape. Embrace the magic of water, and let it guide you on your journey of self-healing and renewal.

CHAPTER 5: THE SCIENCE OF VIBRATION AND FREQUENCY HEALING

* * *

How Sound and Vibrations Affect Brainwaves and Energy

Sound and vibrations are more than mere sensations; they are powerful forces that can transform our brainwaves and energy levels in profound ways. Research has shown that different frequencies can elicit various emotional and physiological responses, making sound a potent tool for healing. When we listen to soothing music or the gentle hum of nature, our brains can shift into states of relaxation and tranquility. These shifts not only enhance our mood but also allow for deeper introspection and connection with our inner selves.

The brain operates on specific wave patterns—gamma, beta, alpha, theta, and delta—each associated with different states of consciousness. Sound and vibrations can influence these brainwave patterns significantly. For instance, binaural beats, which involve presenting two slightly different frequencies to each ear, can induce states ranging from deep relaxation to heightened focus. By harnessing these frequencies, we can effectively tailor our mental state to achieve desired outcomes, whether it's stress relief, increased creativity, or improved concentration.

Moreover, the energy within our bodies responds dynamically to sound vibrations. Traditional practices like sound healing and chanting have long recognized the power of vibration to align and balance our energy centers, or chakras. Each chakra resonates with specific frequencies, and when we expose ourselves to sounds that correspond with these frequencies, we can clear blockages and restore harmony within. This energetic realignment not only enhances our physical well-being but also elevates our spiritual connection, allowing us to access deeper layers of consciousness.

Engaging with sound and vibration doesn't have to be complex or esoteric. Simple practices such as singing, humming, or even using instruments like singing bowls can create transformative experiences. These practices can be easily integrated into daily routines, allowing individuals to cultivate a self-healing environment. By making sound a regular part of our lives, we can promote mental clarity, emotional balance, and overall well-being, transforming our living spaces into sanctuaries of healing.

As we delve deeper into the mysteries of sound and vibration, we unlock the potential to harness these tools for personal transformation. Embracing the profound connection between sound and our internal states can open doors to self-healing and spiritual growth. By exploring this dynamic interplay, we invite a new dimension of wellness into our lives, empowering ourselves to take charge of our healing journey. Let the vibrations guide you, and discover the magic that lies within the frequencies of the universe.

Healing With Binaural Beats, Mantras, and Singing Bowls

* * *

Healing with binaural beats, mantras, and singing bowls opens up a vibrant world of sound that resonates deeply with our inner selves. Each of these modalities taps into the profound healing potential of vibrational frequencies, creating an atmosphere that encourages relaxation, mindfulness, and transformation. Imagine immersing yourself in a cocoon of harmonious sounds that not only soothe your spirit but also promote physical and emotional healing. This subchapter will guide you through these fascinating tools and how they can empower your self-healing journey.

Binaural beats are a remarkable auditory phenomenon that harnesses the power of sound waves to influence brainwave patterns. When two slightly different frequencies are played in each ear, your brain creates a third tone, which can help induce states of relaxation, focus, or meditation. This unique auditory experience can lead to profound shifts in consciousness, making it an effective tool for reducing stress, alleviating anxiety, and enhancing overall well-being. As you engage with binaural beats, you may find yourself entering a meditative state more easily, allowing for deeper introspection and healing.

Mantras, on the other hand, are sacred sounds or phrases that have been used for centuries in various spiritual traditions. The repetition of mantras serves to quiet the mind, center your thoughts, and connect you with your higher self. By chanting or silently repeating a mantra, you create a vibrational frequency that can transform your energy and consciousness. This practice fosters a sense of peace and unity, helping to alleviate emotional blockages and promote self-acceptance. Whether you choose a traditional Sanskrit mantra or create your own, the power of sound can elevate your healing practice significantly.

Singing bowls, often crafted from metal or crystal, produce rich, resonant tones that can envelop you in a sonic embrace. The vibrations created by these bowls penetrate deep into the body, promoting relaxation and releasing tension stored in the muscles and mind. When played during meditation or healing sessions, singing bowls can help balance the chakras and facilitate energy flow throughout the body. The experience is both soothing and invigorating, inviting you to connect with your inner wisdom and intuition. Integrating singing bowls into your healing rituals can enhance your journey towards self-discovery and holistic health.

Combining binaural beats, mantras, and singing bowls creates a powerful triad of sound healing that can elevate your self-care routine. As you explore these modalities, allow yourself to be fully present in the experience, embracing the unique sensations and emotions that arise. Each session can be a new adventure, revealing insights and fostering healing on multiple levels. By immersing yourself in these practices, you not only unlock the secrets of self-healing but also cultivate a deeper connection with your true essence, empowering you on your mystical journey.

Using Tuning Forks and Frequency Therapy for Self-Healing

* * *

Using tuning forks and frequency therapy for self-healing is an exciting journey that opens up a world of vibrational magic and profound transformation. Imagine being able to harness the power of sound to align your energies, release blockages, and promote healing within your mind and body. Tuning forks, with their precise frequencies, can resonate with your being in ways that are both uplifting and deeply restorative. As you explore this technique, you will discover how these simple tools can help you tap into your innate healing abilities.

The beauty of tuning forks lies in their ability to create sound waves that resonate with specific energy centers, or chakras, in the body. Each chakra vibrates at its own unique frequency, and when you apply the corresponding tuning fork, you initiate a harmonious interaction that can help restore balance. This process can be incredibly empowering, as you learn to listen to your body's needs and respond with the healing frequencies it craves. By incorporating this practice into your self-care routine, you can enhance your overall well-being and foster a deeper connection to your inner self.

Frequency therapy is not just about sound; it's about embracing the vibrational essence of life. Every cell in your body has its own frequency, and when these frequencies are disrupted, it can lead to physical and emotional discomfort. Tuning forks serve as a bridge to restore these vibrations, allowing you to release stagnant energy and rejuvenate your spirit. As you begin to experience the calming effects of sound vibrations, you may find that your stress levels decrease, your clarity improves, and a sense of peace envelops you like a warm embrace.

To get started with tuning forks and frequency therapy, you don't need to be an expert. Simply choose a set of tuning forks that resonate with you and set aside a few moments each day for practice. You can strike the forks and hold them near your body or even place them directly on specific areas that need healing. Experiment with different frequencies and notice how they affect your mood and energy levels. This exploration is a delightful journey of self-discovery, where you can uncover new layers of healing and creativity within yourself.

As you integrate tuning forks and frequency therapy into your life, remember that this practice is a celebration of your unique healing journey. Embrace the joy of sound, and allow it to guide you toward greater awareness and understanding of your body's needs. With each session, you'll cultivate a deeper appreciation for the vibrational nature of the universe and your role within it. Let the power of tuning forks elevate your self-healing journey, unlocking the secrets of your true potential and inviting a harmonious balance into your life.

CHAPTER 6: THE ART OF SELF-HEALING THROUGH MEDITATION

* * *

How Meditation Rewires the Brain and Promotes Inner Peace

Meditation is not just a practice; it is a transformative journey that can significantly reshape the architecture of our brains. Research has shown that regular meditation can lead to remarkable changes in brain structure and function. For instance, it enhances the thickness of the prefrontal cortex, which is responsible for higher-order thinking, decision-making, and emotional regulation. These changes contribute to improved focus, greater emotional resilience, and an overall increase in cognitive abilities. By embracing meditation, we actively participate in a process that rewires our neural pathways, fostering a state of mental clarity and emotional stability.

As we delve deeper into meditation, we uncover its profound ability to promote inner peace. The practice encourages a state of mindfulness, allowing us to observe our thoughts without judgment. This non-reactive awareness helps quiet the mind's incessant chatter, creating a tranquil inner landscape. When we cultivate this peaceful state, we can detach from stressors and anxieties that often dominate our daily lives. This shift not only enhances our well-being but also empowers us to respond to challenges with calmness and grace, rather than being swept away by emotional turbulence.

Additionally, the benefits of meditation extend beyond the mind and deeply influence our emotional health. Studies have revealed that consistent meditation practice increases the production of serotonin and dopamine, neurotransmitters that play vital roles in mood regulation. As we meditate, we foster a sense of happiness and contentment, helping to alleviate symptoms of anxiety and depression. The practice becomes a sanctuary where we can recharge our emotional batteries, ensuring that we approach life with a more positive and balanced outlook.

Moreover, meditation fosters a profound connection with ourselves and the world around us. In the stillness of meditation, we often experience moments of clarity and insight, allowing us to understand our true selves better. This self-discovery is crucial for personal growth and healing. As we cultivate self-compassion through meditation, we learn to accept ourselves more fully, letting go of self-criticism and judgment. This nurturing relationship with ourselves lays the foundation for healthier interactions with others, creating a ripple effect of peace and understanding in our communities.

In essence, meditation is a powerful tool for rewiring the brain and promoting inner peace. It enables us to break free from habitual thought patterns that no longer serve us, replacing them with a more adaptive mindset. By integrating meditation into our daily lives, we embrace a holistic approach to self-healing, unlocking the secrets to a more balanced and fulfilling existence. The journey may be challenging, but the rewards of inner peace and enhanced cognitive function are well worth the effort. Embrace this mystic practice, and watch as your life transforms in extraordinary ways.

Guided Visualization Techniques for Energy Healing

* * *

Guided visualization techniques are powerful tools in the realm of energy healing, allowing individuals to harness the mind's innate ability to create profound change. By vividly picturing healing scenarios, practitioners can engage their subconscious, directing energy flows to areas in need of restoration. This practice not only enhances relaxation but also promotes a deep sense of connection with one's inner self, making it an essential component of any self-healing journey.

To begin, one must find a quiet, comfortable space where distractions are minimal. Close your eyes and take several deep breaths, allowing your body to relax completely. Once you feel centered, envision a radiant light surrounding you. This light symbolizes healing energy, and as you breathe in, imagine it filling your body, cleansing it of negativity and tension. Picture this light moving through each chakra, balancing and revitalizing your energy centers. This simple visualization can lead to profound shifts in emotional and physical well-being.

As you become more adept at guided visualization, you

can introduce specific healing intentions. For instance, if you are addressing a particular ailment, visualize the affected area bathed in healing light. Picture the cells rejuvenating, inflammation subsiding, and pain dissipating. Infusing your visualization with emotion can amplify its effectiveness; feel gratitude for your body's ability to heal itself as you visualize. This emotional connection not only deepens the experience but also sends a powerful message to your subconscious, aligning your energy with your desired outcome.

Incorporating sound into your guided visualization can further enhance the experience. Soft music, chanting, or even the sounds of nature can create an immersive environment, elevating the vibrational frequency of your practice. As you visualize, allow the sounds to resonate within you, harmonizing with the healing energy. This multisensory approach can enhance your ability to tap into deeper states of consciousness, facilitating a stronger connection to your healing intentions.

Lastly, make guided visualization a regular part of your self-care routine. Consistency is key in energy healing, and dedicating time each day to this practice can significantly enhance your overall well-being. As you continue to refine your technique, you may find that your ability to visualize and manifest healing becomes more potent, opening doors to new levels of self-discovery and transformation. Embrace this journey with enthusiasm and an open heart, for the power of guided visualization is a gateway to unlocking your true healing potential.

The Connection Between Deep Stillness and Cellular Repair

* * *

In the ever-evolving journey of self-healing, the profound relationship between deep stillness and cellular repair emerges as a cornerstone of holistic wellness. When we enter a state of deep stillness, whether through meditation, breathwork, or simply quieting the mind, we create an environment that is conducive to cellular rejuvenation. This stillness allows our body to shift from a state of stress—which can be detrimental to our health—into a mode of recovery and restoration. The magic lies in the body's ability to heal itself when we provide the right conditions for it to do so.

Deep stillness is not merely the absence of noise or activity; it is a rich, vibrant state of being that invites us to connect with our innermost selves. In this state, our body can activate the parasympathetic nervous system, often referred to as the "rest and digest" system. This activation promotes healing on a cellular level by reducing inflammation, enhancing circulation, and optimizing the immune response. When we become still, we tap into the body's innate wisdom, allowing it to focus its energy on repairing damaged cells, regenerating tissues, and restoring balance.

Moreover, the practice of deep stillness fosters a profound connection between the mind and body. This connection is essential for cellular repair, as mental and emotional states are intricately linked to physical health. Stress, anxiety, and negative emotions can wreak havoc on our cellular integrity, leading to a cascade of health issues. In contrast, embracing stillness cultivates positive emotional states, such as joy and gratitude, which are instrumental in supporting our body's healing processes. The more we practice stillness, the more we reinforce this mind-body connection, empowering our cells to thrive.

The act of entering deep stillness also enhances our awareness of bodily sensations and signals. By tuning into our physical selves, we become more attuned to what our bodies need, whether that's rest, nourishment, or movement. This heightened awareness allows us to respond proactively to our body's signals, creating a feedback loop that supports ongoing cellular repair. As we learn to listen and honor our bodies, we foster an environment where healing can flourish, making each moment of stillness a powerful ally in our self-healing journey.

In conclusion, the connection between deep stillness and cellular repair is a vibrant testament to the power of self-awareness and intentionality. By embracing practices that cultivate deep stillness, we open the door to profound healing at the cellular level. Each moment spent in this state of tranquility not only enhances our physical health but also enriches our spiritual journey. As we unlock the secrets of self-healing through deep stillness, we empower ourselves to embrace a life filled with vitality, resilience, and joy. Let us embark on this transformative path together, celebrating the miraculous capabilities of our bodies and the boundless potential that lies within each of us.

CHAPTER 7: HEALING THROUGH THE POWER OF LIGHT AND COLOR

* * *

The Science of Phototherapy and Light Energy

The science of phototherapy and light energy is an exhilarating intersection of technology and natural healing that opens up a world of possibilities for self-healing. At its core, phototherapy utilizes specific wavelengths of light to stimulate physiological responses in the body, promoting healing and well-being. This awe-inspiring technique leverages the innate power of light, which has been revered across cultures for centuries as a source of life and rejuvenation. With advances in our understanding of light's effects on the human body, we can harness this energy in ways that empower us to take charge of our health and transform our lives.

One of the most fascinating aspects of phototherapy is the role of different wavelengths in eliciting various biological responses. For instance, red and near-infrared light have been shown to penetrate deep into tissues, promoting cellular repair and regeneration. This can significantly aid in healing wounds, reducing inflammation, and alleviating pain. Meanwhile, blue light has garnered attention for its ability to combat acne by targeting bacteria on the skin. Each color of light possesses unique properties, allowing practitioners to customize treatments to target specific ailments. This precision in therapy is a thrilling aspect of phototherapy that underscores its potential in holistic health.

The physiological mechanisms behind phototherapy are equally captivating. When light is absorbed by the skin, it activates photoreceptors within cells, triggering a cascade of biochemical reactions. This process enhances mitochondrial function, leading to increased energy production and improved cellular metabolism. The result? Enhanced healing processes and a boost in overall vitality. The science behind this is not just theoretical; numerous studies have documented the positive effects of light therapy on various health conditions, from chronic pain to mood disorders, making it a promising avenue for self-healing enthusiasts.

Moreover, the accessibility of light therapy devices has democratized healing in ways previously unimaginable. With the advent of at-home light therapy tools, individuals now have the power to incorporate this transformative practice into their daily routines. Whether it's a handheld device for targeted treatment or a full-body panel for systemic benefits, the options are as diverse as the needs of those seeking healing. This accessibility invites everyone to explore the incredible potential of light energy to enhance their well-being, fostering a sense of empowerment and agency over personal health.

As we delve deeper into the world of phototherapy, we begin to unravel the profound connection between light and our physical, emotional, and spiritual well-being. Embracing this scientific approach to healing not only enriches our understanding of the human body but also aligns beautifully with the principles of self-care and holistic health. By integrating light energy into our healing practices, we step into a realm where science meets mysticism, unlocking the secrets to self-healing and nourishing our journey toward optimal health. The possibilities are as bright as the light itself, illuminating a path to wellness that is both exciting and transformational.

Chakra-Based Color Therapy for Emotional Balance

* * *

Chakra-Based Color Therapy harnesses the vibrational energies of colors to promote emotional balance and healing, tapping into the ancient wisdom of chakra systems. Each chakra corresponds to specific colors that resonate with particular emotional states. By understanding and utilizing these colors, we empower ourselves to align our emotional bodies with our higher selves. Imagine the transformative potential of incorporating vibrant hues into your daily life, enhancing your mood and fostering a sense of inner peace.

The root chakra, represented by the color red, is the foundation of our emotional stability and security. When this chakra is balanced, we feel grounded and confident in our ability to navigate life's challenges. However, emotional turmoil or instability can lead to a blockage in this energy center. Engaging with the color red—through clothing, decor, or visualization—can invigorate this chakra, inviting feelings of safety, vitality, and strength. Embrace red in your environment to reawaken your connection to the earth and nurture a sense of belonging.

Moving up the spectrum, the sacral chakra, associated with the color orange, governs our creativity and emotional expression. An imbalance can manifest as emotional numbness or overwhelming feelings. Infusing your life with orange can reignite your passion and joy. Surround yourself with this vibrant hue, whether it's through art, food, or nature, to stimulate your creative energies. Allow the warmth of orange to inspire playful interactions and emotional connections, unlocking the joys of your inner self.

As we rise to the solar plexus chakra, represented by yellow, we tap into our personal power and self-esteem. This chakra is pivotal in our emotional landscape, influencing how we assert ourselves in the world. A deficiency in yellow can lead to feelings of inadequacy or helplessness. Incorporate yellow into your life to cultivate confidence and optimism. Imagine basking in sunlight or decorating your space with cheerful yellow accents; this color can elevate your mood and empower you to shine brightly in every situation you encounter.

The heart chakra, resonating with green, is the center of love, compassion, and emotional healing. When this chakra is open and balanced, we experience deep connections with ourselves and others. However, emotional wounds can create blockages, leading to feelings of loneliness or resentment. Surrounding yourself with green—whether through nature, clothing, or visualization—can facilitate healing and forgiveness. Allow the nurturing energy of green to fill your heart, opening it to love and acceptance, both for yourself and those around you. Embrace this journey of color therapy as a vibrant path to emotional equilibrium and holistic wellness.

Using Sunlight and Artificial Light for Healing

* * *

Sunlight and artificial light are powerful allies in our journey towards self-healing, offering us the opportunity to harness their energy for rejuvenation and wellness. The sun, a timeless source of life, not only brightens our days but also plays a critical role in our physical and mental health. Sunlight stimulates the production of vitamin D, which is essential for maintaining strong bones and a healthy immune system. But beyond its biological benefits, sunlight can elevate our mood and enhance our overall sense of well-being. Taking a few moments each day to bask in the natural light can invigorate our spirits and create a profound connection with the universe.

Incorporating light therapy into our self-healing practices can amplify the benefits of sunlight. This method utilizes artificial light sources to mimic the sun's rays, providing therapeutic effects that can alleviate seasonal affective disorder, improve sleep patterns, and reduce stress. Light therapy devices emit specific wavelengths of light that penetrate the skin and stimulate cellular functions, promoting healing on a deeper level. By creating a dedicated space for this practice, we can transform our environment into a sanctuary of light, where healing energy flows freely, enhancing our mental clarity and emotional resilience.

The colors of light also play a significant role in healing. Each color has its own vibrational frequency and can influence our mood and physical condition. For instance, blue light is known for its calming effects, making it ideal for reducing anxiety and promoting relaxation. Conversely, red light can energize and stimulate circulation, making it perfect for invigorating our bodies during times of fatigue. By consciously selecting the colors of light that surround us, whether through natural sunlight or artificial sources, we can tailor our healing experiences to align with our specific needs and intentions.

Creating rituals that incorporate both sunlight and artificial light can deepen our self-healing practices. Imagine starting your day with a sun salutation, greeting the morning sun while setting intentions for the day ahead. Later, as the sun sets, transitioning to a light therapy session can help you unwind and reflect on the day's experiences. This seamless integration of natural and artificial light can foster a sense of balance and harmony within us, reinforcing our connection to both nature and technology.

Ultimately, the synergy of sunlight and artificial light can unlock new dimensions of healing. By embracing these luminous forces, we not only enhance our physical health but also nurture our emotional and spiritual well-being. The journey of self-healing is illuminated by the light we choose to embrace, allowing us to cultivate a vibrant existence where we can thrive. Let the rays of sunlight and the glow of artificial light be your guides on this transformative path, leading you toward a brighter, healthier future.

CHAPTER 8: THE MIND-BODY CONNECTION IN HEALING

* * *

How Thoughts and Emotions Influence Physical Health

Thoughts and emotions play a pivotal role in shaping our physical health, acting as the bridge between the mind and body. The intricate connection between our mental state and physical well-being has long been recognized in various healing traditions, and modern science continues to uncover the profound impact that emotions can have on our biological systems. When we experience positive emotions such as joy, gratitude, and love, our bodies respond by releasing beneficial hormones and neurotransmitters. This cascade of biochemicals can enhance immunity, reduce inflammation, and promote overall vitality.

Conversely, negative thoughts and emotions can lead to a host of physical ailments. Stress, anxiety, and chronic negative thinking can trigger a cascade of physiological responses that may weaken the immune system, increase inflammation, and contribute to chronic diseases. The body, in its wisdom, reacts to our emotional states, often manifesting these feelings in physical symptoms. For instance, prolonged stress can lead to tension headaches, digestive issues, or even cardiovascular problems. Acknowledging this connection empowers us to take control of our health by cultivating a more positive mental landscape.

Mindfulness practices, such as meditation and deep breathing, can significantly enhance our ability to manage thoughts and emotions. These techniques not only promote relaxation but also foster a greater awareness of our mental patterns. By recognizing and reframing negative thoughts, we can shift our emotional responses, creating a healthier internal environment. Embracing mindfulness allows us to be present with our feelings, transforming them into opportunities for growth rather than sources of distress. As we cultivate this awareness, we can begin to heal our bodies from the inside out.

Another powerful aspect of the mind-body connection is the influence of visualization and positive affirmations. By picturing ourselves in a state of health and vitality, we send signals to our subconscious mind that can enhance our physical well-being. Visualization can be a transformative tool, allowing us to create a mental blueprint of health that the body can follow. Coupling this practice with affirmations reinforces our commitment to self-healing, promoting a sense of agency and positivity that can ripple through our physical body.

Incorporating these principles into our daily lives can lead to profound changes in our health. By nurturing positive thoughts and emotions, we unlock the potential for self-healing that resides within each of us. As we explore the depths of our emotional landscape, we can harness the power of our minds to foster resilience, vitality, and well-being. The journey of self-healing is not just about addressing physical symptoms; it is a holistic endeavor that embraces the interconnectedness of mind, body, and spirit. Embrace this journey with enthusiasm and watch as your health transforms in remarkable ways.

The Role of Neuroplasticity in Rewiring the Brain for Wellness

* * *

Neuroplasticity, the brain's remarkable ability to reorganize itself by forming new neural connections, is a cornerstone of our journey toward wellness. This dynamic process empowers individuals to reshape their thoughts, behaviors, and even emotional responses. Imagine your brain as a living canvas, where each stroke of experience can alter the landscape of your mind. Embracing neuroplasticity means recognizing that no matter your past, you have the power to redefine your future through intentional practice and awareness.

When we engage in mindfulness practices, such as meditation or deep breathing, we actively harness the principles of neuroplasticity. These practices can lead to tangible changes in brain structure and function. Regular meditation, for instance, has been shown to increase the thickness of the prefrontal cortex, the area responsible for decision-making and self-regulation. As we cultivate a sense of calm and presence, we simultaneously build resilience, enabling us to respond to life's challenges with newfound strength and clarity.

Positive affirmations and visualization techniques are also potent tools in this transformative journey. By consistently affirming our worth and visualizing our goals, we can create new neural pathways that support healthier self-perceptions and aspirations. Each time we reinforce these positive beliefs, we weaken the grip of negative thought patterns that may have held us back. This is not merely self-help jargon; it is a scientifically backed approach to rewiring our brains for success and fulfillment.

Moreover, engaging in new learning experiences, whether through acquiring new skills or exploring creative outlets, stimulates neuroplasticity in profound ways. The brain thrives on novelty, and each new challenge we embrace encourages the formation of fresh synapses. This not only enhances cognitive flexibility but also instills a sense of joy and excitement in our lives. As we step out of our comfort zones, we open ourselves to a world of possibilities, inviting growth and transformation.

Ultimately, understanding and embracing neuroplasticity is an invitation to take charge of our mental and emotional well-being. It reminds us that we are not merely passive recipients of our experiences but active creators of our reality. By harnessing the power of neuroplasticity, we can unlock the door to self-healing, crafting a life that resonates with joy, purpose, and fulfillment. The journey to wellness is not just a destination; it is a vibrant and ongoing process of growth and renewal.

Affirmations and Positive Intentions for Cellular Healing

* * *

Affirmations and positive intentions are powerful tools in the realm of cellular healing, serving as catalysts that can transform our physical and emotional well-being. At the core of cellular healing is the understanding that our cells respond to vibrational frequencies, including the thoughts and words we choose to express. By harnessing affirmations, we can consciously shift our inner dialogue to one that promotes healing, vitality, and overall wellness. This energetic shift not only affects our mindset but also communicates profound messages to our cellular structure, encouraging it to align with our healing intentions.

To create effective affirmations for cellular healing, begin by focusing on specific areas of your life that require attention. Whether it's physical ailments, emotional blockages, or mental patterns that no longer serve you, crafting affirmations that resonate deeply with your intentions is crucial. For instance, instead of a general statement like "I am healthy," try something more specific such as "Every cell in my body radiates vitality and harmony." This specificity adds a layer of intention that can enhance the effectiveness of your affirmations, allowing you to connect with your body on a cellular level.

Incorporating positive intentions into your daily routine can amplify the effects of your affirmations. Intentions are more than mere wishes; they are conscious commitments to your healing journey. By setting clear intentions, you create a framework for your affirmations to operate within. For example, if your intention is to foster self-love, you might affirm, "I embrace my true self and nurture my body with love and compassion." This combination of intention and affirmation not only strengthens your resolve but also creates a supportive environment for cellular healing to flourish.

Visualization can further enhance the power of your affirmations and intentions. As you recite your affirmations, imagine the energy of those words permeating every cell in your body, revitalizing and rejuvenating them. Picture a vibrant light enveloping your being, infusing your cells with love, health, and positivity. This practice not only reinforces the messages you are sending to your body but also creates a sense of connection and unity within yourself. The more vividly you can visualize this process, the more impactful your affirmations will become.

Finally, consistency is key in harnessing the full potential of affirmations and positive intentions for cellular healing. Make it a habit to engage with your affirmations daily, whether through morning rituals, meditation, or journaling. Over time, this dedication will lead to profound changes within you. As you nurture your body with positive thoughts and intentions, you will witness a transformation not only in your physical health but also in your emotional and spiritual well-being. Embrace this journey, and allow the magic of affirmations and positive intentions to unlock the secrets of your self-healing.

CHAPTER 9: HERBAL AND NATURAL REMEDIES FOR SELF-HEALING

* * *

The Power of Plant Medicine and Herbal Therapies

The world of plant medicine and herbal therapies is a vibrant tapestry woven from centuries of wisdom and natural healing. As we delve into this remarkable realm, we uncover a treasure trove of remedies that not only nurture the body but also illuminate the spirit. The potent properties of herbs and plants have been revered across cultures, each with its own unique stories and applications. From ancient shamans to modern herbalists, the reverence for these natural healers persists, showcasing their power to facilitate profound transformation and restoration.

One of the most exciting aspects of plant medicine is its ability to address a myriad of ailments, offering a holistic approach that modern medicine often lacks. Herbs such as ashwagandha, known for its adaptogenic properties, can help combat stress and enhance vitality. Meanwhile, chamomile soothes the mind and promotes restful sleep, while turmeric's anti-inflammatory qualities support overall health. These examples illustrate the diverse healing potential nestled within the leaves, roots, and flowers of the plant kingdom. By embracing herbal therapies, we empower ourselves to take an active role in our healing journeys.

Moreover, the synergy found in many herbal combinations amplifies their effectiveness, creating a symphony of healing that resonates deeply within us. Formulas like elderberry and echinacea work together to bolster the immune system, while the combination of ginger and honey can alleviate digestive discomfort. This harmonious interplay not only enhances the therapeutic benefits but also encourages a deeper connection with nature. As we learn to craft our own herbal remedies, we discover the joy of becoming co-creators of our health, tapping into a wellspring of wisdom that has stood the test of time.

The practice of integrating plant medicine into our daily lives fosters mindfulness and intention. When we choose to incorporate herbal teas, tinctures, or infused oils, we engage in a ritual that honors the natural world and our bodies. This conscious choice cultivates awareness, inviting us to listen to our bodies' needs and respond accordingly. As we develop this relationship with plants, we cultivate not only physical healing but also emotional and spiritual growth, transforming our self-care routines into sacred practices that nourish every aspect of our being.

Ultimately, the power of plant medicine and herbal therapies lies in their ability to connect us with the earth and ourselves. In a fast-paced world filled with synthetic solutions, turning to nature offers a refreshing alternative that aligns with our innate healing capabilities. By embracing these ancient practices, we unlock the secrets to self-healing, empowering ourselves to reclaim our health and vitality. Let us embark on this enchanting journey, celebrating the gifts of the earth and the magic of our own resilience.

Adaptogenic Herbs and Their Role in Stress Reduction

* * *

Adaptogenic herbs have emerged as powerful allies in the quest for stress reduction and overall well-being. These remarkable plants possess the unique ability to help the body adapt to stressors, both physical and emotional. By modulating the body's response to stress, adaptogens enable individuals to maintain balance and harmony, paving the way for enhanced resilience and vitality. As we delve into the world of these incredible herbs, you'll discover how they can transform your approach to stress management and self-healing.

One of the most celebrated adaptogens is Ashwagandha, an ancient herb revered in Ayurvedic medicine. Known for its calming effects, Ashwagandha helps lower cortisol levels, the hormone primarily responsible for stress. By incorporating this herb into your daily routine, you can foster a sense of tranquility and focus, allowing you to tackle life's challenges with renewed vigor. Whether enjoyed as a powder in smoothies or taken in supplement form, Ashwagandha is a versatile addition that can support your journey towards emotional and physical balance.

Another fascinating adaptogen is Rhodiola Rosea, often referred to as "golden root." This herb is celebrated for its ability to enhance mental clarity and endurance while simultaneously combating fatigue. Rhodiola works by promoting the production of neurotransmitters that elevate mood, making it an excellent choice for those seeking to uplift their spirits during stressful times. Imagine facing your day with heightened energy and a sharper mind—Rhodiola can help you achieve just that, empowering you to navigate challenges with grace and confidence.

Holy Basil, or Tulsi, is yet another gem in the realm of adaptogens. Known for its profound spiritual significance and health benefits, Holy Basil helps to reduce anxiety and improve emotional resilience. This herb not only calms the mind but also supports the immune system, making it a fantastic ally during periods of high stress. Sipping on a warm cup of Holy Basil tea can become a soothing ritual, allowing you to pause, reflect, and recharge as you embrace a more centered existence.

Incorporating adaptogenic herbs into your lifestyle is a delightful journey of exploration and self-discovery. By understanding their unique properties and effects, you can unlock the secrets to managing stress and enhancing your overall health. As you experiment with these herbs, pay attention to how they resonate with your body and spirit—each individual's experience can vary, making this a personal adventure. Embrace the power of adaptogens and watch as they weave their magic into your daily life, guiding you towards a harmonious balance in the face of life's inevitable stresses.

How to Create Personalized Herbal Healing Rituals

* * *

Creating personalized herbal healing rituals can be an incredibly fulfilling journey that connects you to nature and your own inner wisdom. To begin, it's essential to understand your intentions. Ask yourself what specific healing you seek—whether it's physical, emotional, or spiritual. By clarifying your goals, you lay a solid foundation for your rituals. Embrace the excitement of this exploration! Your intentions will guide you in selecting the right herbs that resonate with your needs, allowing for a richer and more meaningful experience.

Next, immerse yourself in the world of herbs. Each herb carries unique properties and energies that can enhance your healing journey. Research various herbs and their traditional uses; some may promote relaxation, while others may boost immunity or clarify the mind. Create a list of herbs that speak to you, and don't hesitate to follow your intuition. Visit local herbal shops or farmers' markets to connect with the plants personally. Smell their fragrances and feel their textures, as this sensory experience will deepen your connection to them.

Once you have your herbs, it's time to design your ritual. Consider the setting—choose a quiet space where you feel safe and comfortable. Gather your herbs, along with any other elements that inspire you, such as candles, crystals, or music. You might want to create an altar to honor your practice. Arrange items that resonate with your intentions, making it visually appealing and inviting. This setting will enhance the energy of your ritual and help you engage fully in the experience.

As you begin the ritual, take a moment to center yourself. Close your eyes, breathe deeply, and visualize your intentions. You can prepare herbal infusions, tinctures, or use dried herbs in smudging practices. Allow yourself to be creative—combine herbs in ways that feel right to you. As you work with the plants, infuse your energy and love into the process. Speak affirmations or mantras that align with your healing goals, creating a powerful synergy between you and the herbs.

Finally, remember that consistency is key. Make this ritual a part of your routine to deepen your connection with the herbs and the healing energies they provide. Journaling about your experiences can also help you track your progress and insights. Celebrate your successes, no matter how small, and allow your personalized herbal healing rituals to evolve over time. The journey of self-healing through herbal practices not only fosters wellness but also nurtures your spirit, empowering you to embrace your mystical path with joy and enthusiasm.

CHAPTER 10: THE ROLE OF FASTING AND DETOXIFICATION IN SELF-HEALING

* * *

How Intermittent and Extended Fasting Cleanse the Body

Intermittent and extended fasting have emerged as powerful practices for cleansing the body, tapping into ancient wisdom and modern science. When we fast, we initiate a remarkable process that allows our bodies to reset and rejuvenate. This practice not only provides a break from constant digestion but also encourages our bodies to utilize stored energy and eliminate toxins. As we delve into the benefits of fasting, we discover its potential to enhance our overall health and elevate our spiritual well-being.

During fasting, the body enters a state of autophagy, a

natural self-cleaning mechanism where damaged cells are broken down and recycled. This process is akin to a meticulous spring cleaning, where the body discards what no longer serves us, making way for renewal. As we allow this cleansing to occur, we may experience increased mental clarity, heightened energy levels, and a profound sense of connection to our inner selves. The beauty of fasting lies in its ability to promote not only physical purification but also emotional and spiritual growth.

Extended fasting takes this cleansing process to new heights. When we fast for more extended periods, our bodies delve deeper into their reserves, transforming stored fat into energy and releasing an array of beneficial hormones. It is during these extended fasts that we often encounter profound insights and revelations. Many find that the experience allows them to break free from old patterns and habits, fostering a sense of liberation and empowerment. As we navigate this journey, we learn to trust our bodies and embrace the wisdom they hold.

Moreover, fasting can enhance our relationship with food and our bodies. By stepping away from our usual eating routines, we cultivate mindfulness and appreciation for nourishment. We begin to recognize the difference between physical hunger and emotional cravings, allowing us to make more conscious choices post-fast. This newfound awareness not only promotes healthier eating habits but also fosters self-love and acceptance, essential components of the self-healing journey.

Incorporating intermittent and extended fasting into our lives can be a transformative experience, unlocking the door to vibrant health and spiritual awakening. As we embark on this path, we embrace the potential for deep healing and self-discovery. With each fast, we cleanse not just our bodies but also our minds and spirits, paving the way for a more harmonious existence. Let us celebrate the magic of fasting and the incredible journey it offers toward self-healing and personal empowerment.

The Science of Cellular Autophagy and Regeneration

* * *

Cellular autophagy is a fascinating process that acts as the body's internal recycling system. It allows cells to break down and remove damaged components, ensuring they operate at peak efficiency. This remarkable mechanism is not merely a survival tactic; it plays a crucial role in maintaining cellular health and overall vitality. When we engage in practices that stimulate autophagy, we unlock the potential for renewal and rejuvenation, paving the way for profound self-healing experiences.

The science behind autophagy is rooted in the intricate dance of cellular processes. During this phenomenon, cells identify dysfunctional proteins and organelles, encapsulating them in double-membraned vesicles known as autophagosomes. These vesicles then fuse with lysosomes, where the contents are degraded and recycled. This process not only clears out cellular debris but also provides essential building blocks for new, healthy cellular structures. By harnessing the power of autophagy, we can significantly enhance our body's ability to heal from within.

Regeneration, closely linked to autophagy, is the body's natural response to injury and stress. When cells undergo stress, whether from environmental factors, toxins, or lifestyle choices, autophagy kicks into high gear, promoting cellular repair and regeneration. This regenerative capacity is vital for maintaining homeostasis and responding to the challenges we face daily. Practices such as fasting, exercise, and specific dietary choices can enhance autophagy, allowing us to tap into our inherent healing capabilities and foster resilience against disease.

The benefits of stimulating autophagy extend beyond mere cellular maintenance; they encompass a holistic approach to self-healing. Enhanced autophagy has been linked to improved metabolic health, reduced inflammation, and even increased longevity. By incorporating mindful practices that promote autophagy into our daily routines, we not only support our physical health but also cultivate a deeper connection to our bodies. This awareness fosters a sense of empowerment, as we recognize our ability to influence our well-being through conscious choices.

As we delve deeper into the science of cellular autophagy and regeneration, it becomes clear that these processes are integral to our self-healing journey. Embracing the principles of autophagy can lead to a transformative experience, unlocking the secrets to vibrant health and vitality. By understanding and engaging with our body's natural mechanisms, we can create a synergy between science and mysticism, allowing us to thrive in harmony with ourselves and the world around us.

Best Detox Practices for Mind, Body, and Spirit

* * *

Detoxifying the mind, body, and spirit is an essential practice in the journey of self-healing. To truly thrive, one must engage in holistic cleansing that transcends mere physical detoxification. Begin by embracing mindfulness techniques that foster clarity and focus. Meditation serves as a powerful tool to clear mental clutter, allowing thoughts to settle like sediment in a jar of water. Set aside a few minutes each day to immerse yourself in stillness, breathing deeply as you visualize negativity leaving your body with each exhale. This practice not only enhances mental clarity but also cultivates a profound connection to your inner self, paving the way for spiritual renewal.

Equally important is the physical aspect of detoxification. Cleanse your body with nutrient-rich foods that promote vitality and energy. Incorporate fresh fruits, vegetables, and whole grains into your diet while eliminating processed foods and artificial additives. Hydration is paramount, so drink plenty of water infused with lemon or herbs to boost your body's natural detox processes. Consider engaging in activities like yoga or brisk walking to stimulate circulation and sweat out toxins. The synergy between nourishing your body and engaging in physical movement creates a vibrant energy flow, enhancing your overall well-being.

Detoxing the spirit is perhaps the most profound and often overlooked element of holistic cleansing. Engage in activities that resonate with your soul, whether that be journaling, painting, or connecting with nature. These creative outlets allow you to express your innermost feelings and release emotional blockages. Furthermore, consider practicing gratitude daily. Reflect on the blessings in your life, no matter how small they may seem. This simple act shifts your focus from what is lacking to what is abundant, fostering a positive mindset that rejuvenates the spirit.

Additionally, surrounding yourself with positive energy is crucial for a successful detox. Evaluate your relationships and environments, seeking to distance yourself from negativity and toxicity. Create a sacred space in your home filled with uplifting items such as crystals, candles, or meaningful artwork. This sanctuary becomes a retreat for your mind, body, and spirit, promoting healing and tranquility. Engage with like-minded individuals who support your journey, as community plays a vital role in sustaining motivation and encouragement.

Finally, remember that detoxification is a continuous journey. Regularly revisit and refine your practices to align with your evolving needs. Embrace seasonal detoxes that correspond with the cycles of nature, allowing your body and spirit to sync with the rhythms of the earth. Celebrate your progress, no matter how small, and honor yourself for taking the steps toward holistic wellness. By committing to these best detox practices, you unlock the secrets of self-healing, paving the way for a vibrant life filled with harmony, joy, and purpose.

CHAPTER 11: ENERGY HEALING TECHNIQUES FOR DEEP RESTORATION

* * *

The Science of Reiki, Qi Gong, and Pranic Healing

The practice of energy healing has fascinated cultures around the globe for centuries, and the science behind modalities like Reiki, Qi Gong, and Pranic Healing offers a compelling glimpse into the interconnectedness of body, mind, and spirit. At its core, these practices are rooted in the understanding that our bodies are not just physical entities but vibrant systems of energy. This energetic perspective transcends traditional Western medicine, inviting us to explore how life force energy, known as "ki" in Reiki, "qi" in Qi Gong, and "prana" in Pranic Healing, can be harnessed for healing and transformation.

Reiki involves channeling universal life force energy through the practitioner's hands to the recipient, promoting relaxation and healing on multiple levels. Scientific studies have begun to validate the efficacy of Reiki, showing reductions in stress, anxiety, and pain among those who receive it. This process isn't just about physical healing; it also fosters emotional and spiritual balance. Through Reiki, practitioners create a sacred space where individuals can release blockages and restore harmony, emphasizing the mind-body connection and the profound impact of intention in the healing process.

Qi Gong, an ancient Chinese practice, combines movement, meditation, and breath control to cultivate and balance qi within the body. Research indicates that regular practice of Qi Gong can enhance immune function, improve circulation, and reduce chronic pain. The beauty of Qi Gong lies in its accessibility; anyone can engage in this practice, regardless of age or physical ability. As practitioners learn to flow with their breath and movement, they become attuned to the natural rhythms of their bodies, leading to increased vitality and a deeper sense of inner peace.

Pranic Healing takes a unique approach by focusing on the energy body, or aura, to cleanse and energize it. This technique involves scanning the body for imbalances, removing stagnant energy, and replenishing it with fresh prana. Scientific exploration into energy fields has shown that our emotional and physical states can be influenced by the health of our energy bodies. As Pranic Healing practitioners develop their sensitivity to these energy shifts, they empower individuals to take charge of their own healing journeys, fostering self-awareness and personal responsibility in the healing process.

The synthesis of Reiki, Qi Gong, and Pranic Healing illustrates a powerful understanding of holistic health. Each modality offers its unique insights and techniques, but they all converge on the fundamental principle that we are all energetic beings capable of profound self-healing. By embracing these practices, individuals can unlock their innate potential, navigate their healing journeys with confidence, and discover a pathway to vibrant health and well-being. This exploration into the science of these modalities not only enriches our understanding but also ignites a passion for holistic healing that can transform lives.

How to Activate and Direct Healing Energy Within Yourself

* * *

Activating and directing healing energy within yourself is an empowering and transformative experience. It begins with a deep sense of awareness, recognizing that the power to heal lies within you. The first step is to cultivate a quiet mind through practices like meditation or deep breathing. Find a comfortable space where you can sit or lie down without distractions. Close your eyes, focus on your breath, and allow your thoughts to settle like leaves floating on a serene pond. This internal stillness creates a fertile ground for healing energy to emerge.

Once you have established this calm state, visualize the energy within you. Picture it as a warm, glowing light, radiating from your core and expanding outward. This light can take on any color you resonate with; many find green or gold symbolically linked to healing. As you breathe in deeply, imagine this energy growing brighter and more vibrant, filling your body with warmth and positivity. Feel it pulsing through every cell, every organ, and every muscle, washing away tension, negativity, and pain. Embrace this sensation; it is a reminder of your innate ability to heal.

Next, direct this energy toward specific areas needing attention. You might focus on physical ailments, emotional wounds, or even spiritual imbalances. Visualize the healing light streaming into these areas, dissolving blockages and restoring balance. You can use affirmations or mantras to reinforce your intention. Phrases like "I am whole" or "I am healing" can amplify the energy flow. Trust in the process and allow your intuition to guide you; your body knows where it needs healing the most.

Incorporating movement can also enhance the activation

of healing energy. Engage in gentle yoga, tai chi, or even a simple dance to connect your body and spirit. As you move, imagine the energy swirling and flowing freely throughout your being. This physical expression not only activates the energy but also encourages it to flow more freely. Remember, healing is not merely a passive experience; it is a dynamic journey that involves active participation and joy.

Finally, integrate the practice of gratitude into your healing routine. After each session, take a moment to express thanks for the energy you have activated and the healing you have experienced. Gratitude not only amplifies your healing energy but also cultivates a positive mindset, allowing you to attract even more healing into your life. As you continue to practice activating and directing healing energy, you will discover new depths of your potential and a profound connection to your inner self, unlocking the secrets of self-healing in the most exhilarating ways.

Using Hands-on and Distant Healing for Self-Renewal

* * *

Using hands-on and distant healing for self-renewal opens up a world of possibilities for transformation and revitalization. Imagine tapping into the profound energy that surrounds you, channeling it to heal not just your body, but your spirit and mind as well. Hands-on healing techniques, such as Reiki or therapeutic touch, allow practitioners to create a powerful connection with their own energy field and that of others. This tangible interaction can bring about immediate relief from stress, anxiety, and physical discomfort, offering a refreshing sense of rejuvenation. As you engage in these practices, you'll discover the vibrant energy that flows through you, igniting a spark of self-renewal that can change your life.

Distant healing, on the other hand, takes this experience to a whole new level. Imagine being able to send or receive healing energy across time and space, breaking the barriers that often limit our ability to heal. Techniques such as visualization and intention-setting allow you to connect with others energetically, facilitating healing even when you're physically apart. This practice empowers you to reach beyond your immediate surroundings, extending your influence and care to loved ones or even those in need around the globe. As you explore distant healing, you'll find that the power of intention can create ripples of healing energy that resonate far and wide.

Incorporating both hands-on and distant healing into your self-care routine can lead to profound self-renewal. Start by integrating hands-on techniques into your daily life. Create a sacred space where you can practice self-healing, perhaps through meditation, breathwork, or energy alignment exercises. Allow yourself to fully immerse in the experience, feeling the energy coursing through your body as you release tension and invite relaxation. As you cultivate this practice, notice the shifts in your physical and emotional state; you may find clarity, peace, and an invigorated sense of purpose blossoming within you.

Next, embrace the power of distant healing as a complementary technique. Set aside time each week to connect with loved ones or even send healing energy to yourself from a distance. You can visualize sending light and love to someone who needs it, or even to past experiences that require healing. The beauty of distant healing lies in its ability to transcend limitations, allowing you to engage with your inner energy and the energy of others in a way that feels expansive and liberating. This practice not only nurtures your own healing journey but also fosters a sense of interconnectedness with the world around you.

Ultimately, the journey of self-renewal through hands-on

and distant healing is one of empowerment and discovery. As you learn to harness these techniques, you'll find that you possess the ability to nurture your own well-being and support those around you. Each session of hands-on healing or distant connection is an opportunity for growth, healing, and transformation. Embrace this journey with enthusiasm, and watch as it unfolds new paths of possibility, inviting you to step into your highest potential and live a life filled with vitality and joy.

CHAPTER 12: SACRED RITUALS AND SPIRITUAL PRACTICES FOR HEALING

* * *

The Role of Rituals in Strengthening Mind-Body Awareness

Rituals serve as powerful tools for enhancing mind-body awareness, offering a structured framework within which individuals can explore their inner selves. By engaging in specific, repeated actions, we create a bridge between our thoughts and physical sensations, deepening our understanding of how they interconnect. This dynamic interplay is essential for self-healing, as it allows us to cultivate a heightened state of mindfulness. Whether it's through meditation, yoga, or simple daily routines, rituals invite us to pause, reflect, and truly tune into our bodies, paving the way for transformative experiences.

The beauty of rituals lies in their versatility. Each person can tailor them to suit their unique needs and preferences, making the practice deeply personal and meaningful. From lighting a candle to signify the beginning of a meditation session to performing a series of stretches that honor our bodies, these actions reinforce our intention to connect with ourselves. As we engage in these rituals, we not only become more aware of our physical presence but also foster a sense of safety and comfort within. This nurturing environment encourages us to explore our emotions freely, leading to profound self-discovery and healing.

Moreover, rituals often involve the use of symbols and elements that resonate with us on a deeper level. Incorporating items like crystals, essential oils, or sacred texts can enhance our experience, as they serve as tangible reminders of our intentions. These elements help anchor our focus, allowing our minds to settle while our bodies engage in the ritual. As we immerse ourselves in these practices, we learn to listen to our bodies' signals more attentively, recognizing patterns of tension or discomfort that may have previously gone unnoticed. Such awareness is crucial for addressing underlying issues and fostering holistic well-being.

Rituals also create a sense of community and shared experience, which can be incredibly healing. Engaging in group rituals, whether in a class or a gathering, amplifies the energy of the practice, allowing participants to support one another on their journeys. This collective experience fosters connection, reminding us that we are not alone in our struggles. The shared intention of self-healing creates a powerful resonance, enhancing our mind-body awareness as we collectively explore the depths of our consciousness. In this way, rituals become a catalyst for personal and communal transformation.

In conclusion, the role of rituals in strengthening mind-body awareness is undeniable. As we embrace these sacred practices, we open ourselves to a world of self-discovery and healing. The consistency and intention behind rituals not only deepen our connection to ourselves but also empower us to face challenges with resilience and grace. By weaving rituals into the fabric of our daily lives, we embark on a journey that nurtures our spirit, strengthens our bodies, and enhances our overall well-being. Let us celebrate the magic of rituals and harness their potential to unlock the secrets of self-healing.

Sacred Smudging, Prayer, and Energy Clearing Practices

* * *

Sacred smudging, prayer, and energy clearing practices are powerful rituals that connect us to the universe's abundant healing energies. These practices have been embraced across various cultures for centuries, serving as a bridge between the spiritual and physical realms. When we engage in smudging, we purify not only our surroundings but also our inner selves, creating an environment ripe for healing and transformation. The aromatic smoke of sacred herbs like sage, sweetgrass, and palo santo carries intentions, inviting clarity and balance into our lives.

As we embark on this journey of self-healing, let us explore the art of smudging. This time-honored practice involves lighting dried herbs and allowing their fragrant smoke to envelop us. The act of smudging is more than a ritual; it is a declaration of our intent to release negativity and invite positive energy. By moving the smoke around our bodies and spaces, we create a sacred atmosphere where healing can flourish. Imagine the gentle tendrils of smoke swirling around you, each curl carrying away stress and anxiety, leaving behind a sense of peace and clarity.

Prayer, too, is a vital component of our energy-clearing practices. It is a personal, intimate connection to the divine, a moment of surrender where we express our deepest desires and fears. Whether spoken aloud or whispered in silence, prayer serves as a conduit for healing energy. Invoking higher powers or the universe at large, we invite guidance and support in our quest for wellness. Each word becomes a vessel of intention, amplifying our desires and aligning our energies with the universal flow. The power of prayer lies not only in the words we choose but in the sincerity of our hearts and the clarity of our intentions.

Energy clearing practices extend beyond smudging and prayer; they encompass a variety of techniques designed to restore harmony within and around us. Visualization, sound healing, and crystal work are just a few examples of how we can engage with the energy around us. Visualizing light surrounding us as we breathe deeply can help wash away stagnant energy, while the soothing sounds of singing bowls or chimes resonate to shift our vibrations. Incorporating crystals into our routines can enhance our energy clearing, as each stone holds unique properties to support healing. The combination of these elements creates a holistic approach to our well-being, allowing us to tap into the vibrational frequencies that promote healing.

As we integrate sacred smudging, prayer, and energy clearing practices into our daily lives, we unlock profound potential for self-healing. These rituals empower us to take charge of our wellness journey, fostering a sense of connection to ourselves, each other, and the universe. By cultivating a sacred space filled with intention, we allow healing energies to flow freely, transforming our lives one ritual at a time. Embrace these practices wholeheartedly, and watch as they illuminate your path, guiding you toward greater peace, clarity, and empowerment on your journey of self-discovery.

Creating a Personal Healing Sanctuary at Home

* * *

Creating a personal healing sanctuary at home is a transformative journey that invites peace, clarity, and rejuvenation into your life. Imagine a space that resonates with your soul, where every element is carefully chosen to support your healing process. This sanctuary can be a corner of a room, a dedicated room, or even an outdoor space—wherever you feel most at ease. The beauty of this endeavor lies in its personal nature; it is entirely up to you to infuse your sanctuary with elements that inspire tranquility and uplift your spirit.

To begin, consider the environment in which you want to create this sacred space. Choose a location in your home that feels comfortable and inviting. It could be by a window where sunlight streams in, or a quiet nook away from distractions. Once you have identified the perfect spot, think about the colors that soothe your mind and spirit. Soft hues, such as gentle blues, greens, or warm earth tones, can create an atmosphere of calm. Paint the walls or add decor that reflects these colors to establish a harmonious backdrop for your sanctuary.

Next, focus on the sensory elements that will enhance your experience. Incorporate textures that feel good to the touch, such as soft cushions, cozy blankets, and natural materials like wood or stone. Introduce scents that promote relaxation and healing—essential oils, incense, or fresh flowers can work wonders. Consider the sounds that calm you; whether it's soft music, nature sounds, or even silence, ensure your sanctuary can envelop you in an audio embrace that supports your journey. Every detail contributes to a sensory oasis that invites you to unwind and reconnect with yourself.

As you design your sanctuary, think about the practices that resonate with your healing journey. This could include a meditation corner with comfortable seating and cushions, a small altar featuring items that hold personal significance, or even a bookshelf filled with inspiring literature. Incorporate tools that aid in your self-healing, such as crystals, journals, or art supplies. Allow your creativity to flow and express your unique vision. Your sanctuary should be a reflection of your inner self, a place where you can explore your thoughts, feelings, and aspirations freely.

Finally, make a commitment to regularly spend time in your healing sanctuary. Consistency is key to reaping the benefits of this sacred space. Whether it's daily meditation, journaling, or simply sitting in silence, carve out moments in your routine to nurture your spirit. Allow this sanctuary to evolve as you grow, welcoming new elements that resonate with your journey. As you cultivate this personal haven, you will find that it becomes a powerful tool for self-discovery and healing, a space where you can unlock the secrets within and flourish on your path to well-being.

CHAPTER 13: MOVEMENT AS MEDICINE – YOGA, TAI CHI, AND QI GONG

* * *

How Conscious Movement Unlocks Stagnant Energy

Conscious movement is an empowering practice that acts as a catalyst for unlocking stagnant energy within our bodies. As we navigate through life, we often accumulate tension and blockages that hinder the free flow of our vital energy. Engaging in conscious movement, whether through yoga, dance, or mindful walking, allows us to reconnect with our physical selves, fostering a sense of awareness that can reveal and release these energetic blockages. By intentionally moving our bodies, we can tap into the profound wisdom they hold and facilitate a transformative healing process.

When we engage in conscious movement, we bring our attention to the sensations within our bodies. This heightened awareness helps us identify areas where energy feels stuck or stagnant. As we breathe deeply and move mindfully, we create space for these areas to open up. The act of movement itself becomes a form of communication with our bodies. It signals to us where we may be holding onto stress, fear, or unresolved emotions. By acknowledging these sensations and allowing ourselves to move through them, we initiate a release that can lead to profound emotional and physical healing.

Moreover, conscious movement encourages the flow of prana, or life force energy, throughout our bodies. Each deliberate action we take, each stretch and bend, acts like a gentle massage for our internal systems. This not only promotes circulation but also enhances our connection to the earth and the present moment. As we engage in this practice, we cultivate a state of flow that can unlock creativity, clarity, and inspiration. The more we practice conscious movement, the more adept we become at recognizing the subtle shifts in our energy, allowing us to respond dynamically to our inner needs.

Incorporating conscious movement into our daily lives can also foster a deeper sense of self-acceptance and love. As we move with intention, we learn to appreciate our bodies for their capabilities rather than their limitations. This shift in perspective can be liberating, as it empowers us to embrace our unique journey and celebrate the progress we make along the way. The more we honor our bodies through conscious movement, the more we cultivate a nurturing relationship with ourselves, which is essential for unlocking stagnant energy.

Ultimately, how conscious movement unlocks stagnant energy is a journey of self-discovery and healing. It invites us to explore the intricate connections between our physical, emotional, and spiritual selves. By committing to this practice, we open ourselves to the possibility of transformation and renewal. With every conscious movement, we step closer to our true essence, releasing what no longer serves us and welcoming the vibrant energy that resides within. Embrace this journey, and watch how the act of moving with intention can lead to profound shifts in your life.

The Healing Science of Flow, Posture, and Breath Coordination

* * *

The healing science of flow, posture, and breath coordination is a captivating journey into the depths of our being. Imagine a state where your body moves gracefully, your breath flows effortlessly, and your mind is a serene lake reflecting the beauty of the world around you. This harmonious trifecta can unlock incredible healing potential, transforming not only your physical health but also your emotional and spiritual well-being. By understanding and practicing the art of flow, posture, and breath, you can access a profound state of self-healing that empowers you to thrive in all aspects of life.

Flow is the essence of movement, the rhythm that connects your mind and body. When you engage in activities that promote flow, such as yoga, dance, or tai chi, you tap into a natural state of being where time seems to dissolve and you become one with the present moment. This state has been scientifically shown to reduce stress and anxiety, boost creativity, and enhance overall well-being. Embracing flow not only allows you to experience joy in movement but also fosters a deeper connection with your inner self, paving the way for remarkable healing experiences.

Posture is more than just how you sit or stand; it is a powerful reflection of your mental and emotional state. Proper posture aligns your body and allows energy to flow freely throughout your system. When you maintain an open and confident posture, you send signals to your brain that promote feelings of empowerment and positivity. Conversely, slouched or closed positions can hinder energy flow and contribute to feelings of lethargy or sadness. By cultivating awareness of your posture and making intentional adjustments, you can significantly enhance your mood and overall health, allowing the healing process to unfold naturally.

Breath coordination is the final piece of this healing puzzle. Conscious breathing techniques can dramatically influence your physical and emotional state. When you focus on your breath, you engage the parasympathetic nervous system, which promotes relaxation and reduces stress. Techniques such as deep abdominal breathing or rhythmic breathing patterns can enhance oxygen flow to your cells, invigorate your body, and clear your mind. By synchronizing your breath with movement and posture, you create a powerful synergy that not only revitalizes your physical body but also elevates your spirit, creating a truly transformative experience.

Together, flow, posture, and breath coordination form a holistic approach to self-healing that is both accessible and profoundly effective. Embracing these elements in your daily life opens the door to a vibrant existence filled with energy, clarity, and peace. As you explore these practices, you will discover the incredible potential that lies within you, empowering you to navigate life's challenges with grace and resilience. Dive into this healing science, and unlock the secrets that will lead you to a healthier, happier, and more fulfilling life.

Daily Movement Practices for Longevity and Vitality

* * *

Daily movement practices are vital for cultivating longevity and vitality, serving as a bridge between the physical body and the profound energy within. Engaging in consistent movement not only enhances physical fitness but also nourishes the spirit, allowing us to connect deeply with ourselves. Imagine waking up each day, feeling energized and ready to embrace the world, simply by integrating movement into your routine. Whether through dance, walking, yoga, or tai chi, each practice offers a unique pathway to unlocking your potential for self-healing and vibrant living.

One of the most accessible forms of movement is walking, a practice that invites us to connect with our surroundings and clear our minds. Stepping outside for a brisk walk not only elevates our heart rate but also opens our senses to the beauty of nature. The rhythmic motion of walking can be meditative, allowing thoughts to drift away while fostering clarity and creativity. As we immerse ourselves in the sights and sounds around us, we also cultivate gratitude and mindfulness, essential ingredients for a healthy, fulfilled life.

Yoga is another powerful daily movement practice that promotes longevity and vitality. With its roots in ancient wisdom, yoga harmonizes the body, mind, and spirit, making it an ideal practice for self-healing. Each pose invites us to explore our physical limitations while encouraging flexibility and strength. Breathwork, an integral part of yoga, enhances our life force, rejuvenating our energy levels and calming our minds. Dedicating even a few minutes daily to yoga can yield profound benefits, creating a sanctuary within ourselves that radiates peace and vitality.

Dance, often overlooked as a form of exercise, is also a joyous way to move our bodies and connect with our essence. Whether it's free-form dancing in your living room or taking a structured class, the act of dancing ignites our creativity and lifts our spirits. It encourages us to express ourselves freely and sheds inhibitions, allowing for a deeper connection to our emotions. This playful movement not only strengthens our bodies but also reinvigorates our souls, paving the way for a life filled with vitality and enthusiasm.

Lastly, incorporating practices like tai chi and qigong into your daily routine can significantly enhance your overall health and longevity. These ancient martial arts focus on slow, deliberate movements and deep breathing, promoting balance, flexibility, and mental clarity. As you engage in these gentle practices, you will notice a profound shift in your energy, encouraging the flow of vital life force throughout your body. By embracing these daily movement practices, you open the door to a life brimming with vitality, resilience, and joyful self-discovery, unlocking the true potential of your healing journey.

CHAPTER 14: DREAMWORK AND THE SUBCONSCIOUS MIND IN HEALING

* * *

How Dreams Reveal Emotional and Energetic Imbalances

Dreams serve as a powerful window into our subconscious, revealing the emotional and energetic imbalances that may be lurking beneath the surface. Each night, when we drift into the realm of sleep, our minds become a canvas for the vivid imagery of our inner world. These dreamscapes are not random; they are rich with symbolism and messages that can illuminate our emotional states. By paying close attention to our dreams, we can uncover hidden feelings, unresolved conflicts, and energetic blockages that may be affecting our overall well-being.

When we analyze our dreams, we often discover recurring themes or symbols that point directly to our emotional health. For instance, dreaming of being chased may indicate feelings of anxiety or avoidance in waking life. Such dreams can act as a mirror, reflecting our fears and insecurities, urging us to confront what we might be neglecting. By engaging with these dreams through journaling or conversation, we create an opportunity for self-reflection and healing. This process allows us to transform our fears into actionable insights, paving the way for emotional resilience.

Energetic imbalances often manifest in our dreams as peculiar scenarios or intense emotions. A dream of being trapped might signal stagnation in our lives, suggesting that we are not fully expressing ourselves or pursuing our passions. Recognizing these patterns is crucial, as they highlight areas where we may need to release pent-up energy or make significant changes. Engaging in practices such as meditation or energy healing can help restore balance, allowing us to harmonize our inner and outer worlds. Dreams become a catalyst for transformation, guiding us toward a more vibrant existence.

Moreover, dreams can also reveal the connections between our emotional state and our physical health. The mind-body connection is profound, and when we experience emotional turmoil, it can manifest as physical symptoms. Dreaming of illness or discomfort may point to repressed emotions that require attention. By interpreting these dreams, we can gain insights into the areas of our lives that need healing, encouraging us to address not only our emotional pain but also any physical manifestations it may have created. This holistic approach promotes overall wellness and fosters a deeper understanding of our mind-body connection.

Ultimately, our dreams are a treasure trove of guidance and wisdom, offering us a unique perspective on our emotional and energetic imbalances. By embracing the messages they convey, we empower ourselves to take charge of our healing journey. Each dream is an invitation to explore our inner landscape, confront our fears, and align our energies. As we delve deeper into the mysterious world of dreams, we unlock the potential for profound transformation, leading us toward a more harmonious and fulfilling life. The journey of self-discovery through dream analysis is not only enlightening but also exhilarating, making it an essential practice in the pursuit of self-healing.

Lucid Dreaming as a Tool for Self-Healing

* * *

Lucid dreaming serves as a fascinating gateway to self-healing, enabling individuals to tap into their subconscious mind and access profound insights. As you become aware that you are dreaming, a unique opportunity arises to confront fears, explore emotions, and heal psychological wounds. The beauty of lucid dreaming lies in its potential to transform nightmares into empowering experiences. Instead of being paralyzed by fear, you can take control, rewrite the narrative, and emerge from the dream with a renewed sense of strength and clarity.

Engaging in lucid dreaming encourages a deep level of introspection. By actively participating in your dreams, you can connect with aspects of yourself that may be hidden during waking hours. This self-exploration allows for the examination of unresolved issues and emotional baggage that might otherwise remain buried. Embracing this level of consciousness can lead to profound revelations about personal challenges, fostering understanding and acceptance. As these insights surface, you pave the way for healing, allowing the mind to release what no longer serves you.

Moreover, lucid dreaming can serve as a powerful tool

for overcoming anxiety and stress. In a controlled dream environment, you can practice coping strategies and visualize solutions to real-life problems. Whether it's rehearsing for a difficult conversation or simply cultivating a sense of peace, the mind's ability to simulate experiences can significantly impact your waking life. By facing challenges within the dream state, you can diminish their power, allowing for a more serene and confident approach to life's hurdles.

In addition to psychological healing, lucid dreaming can also enhance physical well-being. Research suggests that our mental state significantly influences our physical health. By engaging in lucid dreams, you can visualize healing processes, whether it's imagining your body free of illness or visualizing energy flowing through you. This mental imagery can bolster the body's natural healing mechanisms, contributing to an overall sense of vitality. Through these dream experiences, individuals often report improvements in physical ailments, highlighting the mind-body connection that is so crucial to holistic healing.

Finally, the practice of lucid dreaming cultivates a sense of empowerment and agency in one's life. It fosters the belief that you can shape your reality, both in dreams and waking life. This newfound confidence can extend beyond the dream realm, encouraging you to pursue personal goals, confront challenges, and embrace change. As you harness the power of lucid dreaming, you not only embark on a journey of self-discovery but also unlock the potential for transformative healing. By embracing this mystical tool, you open the door to a world where the possibilities for growth and rejuvenation are limitless.

Tapping Into the Wisdom of the Subconscious Through Dreams

* * *

Tapping into the wisdom of the subconscious through dreams is an exhilarating journey into the depths of your own psyche. Dreams are not just random images or fleeting thoughts; they are gateways to a profound understanding of ourselves. As we drift into sleep, our subconscious mind takes the reins, weaving together the threads of our daily experiences, fears, desires, and unresolved issues. By actively engaging with our dreams, we can uncover insights that can lead to powerful self-healing and transformation.

The first step in harnessing the wisdom of your dreams is to cultivate awareness. Keep a dream journal by your bedside and jot down your dreams as soon as you wake up. This practice not only helps you remember your dreams more vividly, but it also creates a sacred space for reflection. As you revisit your entries, patterns and symbols may emerge, revealing hidden themes in your life. These recurring motifs are often the key to unlocking deeper understanding and self-awareness, guiding you toward the areas of your life that need healing.

Interpreting dreams can be both an art and a science. Each dream is a unique tapestry woven from your personal experiences and emotions, and while there are many universal symbols, the meaning of a dream can vary for each individual. Embrace the process of interpretation by asking yourself questions about the dream's imagery and emotions. What feelings did you experience? What issues were brought to light? Engaging with these questions allows your subconscious to communicate its wisdom, offering you clarity and direction as you navigate your healing journey.

In addition to personal reflection, consider incorporating creative practices into your dream exploration. Art, writing, or even movement can serve as powerful tools to express the emotions and insights that arise from your dreams. Allow your creative instincts to flow freely, and you may find that the act of creation deepens your understanding of the messages from your subconscious. This vibrant exchange can lead to breakthroughs that propel you further on your path to self-healing.

Finally, don't forget the power of community in this process. Sharing your dreams with trusted friends or a dream group can provide fresh perspectives and insights that you might not see on your own. Engaging in discussions about dreams can foster a sense of connection and support, reinforcing the idea that you are not alone on this journey. Together, you can explore the rich landscape of your dreams, helping each other unlock the secrets that will lead to greater self-awareness and healing. Embrace the adventure of tapping into the wisdom of your subconscious through dreams, and watch as your life transforms in remarkable ways.

CHAPTER 15: MANIFESTATION AND THE LAW OF HEALING INTENTIONS

* * *

How the Law of Attraction Works in Healing

The Law of Attraction is an empowering principle that suggests our thoughts and emotions can significantly influence our reality, including our health and well-being. When we embrace this law in the context of healing, we begin to understand that our mindset and energy play crucial roles in the healing process. By focusing on positive thoughts and visualizations, we can align ourselves with the vibrations of health and vitality, effectively drawing them into our lives. This transformative approach allows us to take an active role in our healing journey, reinforcing the idea that we are not merely passive recipients of circumstances but powerful creators of our own reality.

As we harness the Law of Attraction, it's essential to cultivate a mindset that is conducive to healing. This involves letting go of limiting beliefs and negative thought patterns that may have been ingrained in us over time. Replacing these with affirmations of health, resilience, and positivity can create a ripple effect throughout our lives. Each time we affirm our ability to heal, we reinforce a powerful signal to the universe that we are ready to receive abundance, joy, and well-being. This shift in perspective not only fosters a more positive emotional state but also opens us up to new possibilities for healing that we may not have considered before.

Visualization is a potent tool within the framework of the Law of Attraction, particularly in healing. Picture your body bathed in radiant health, filled with vibrant energy, and free from ailments. By vividly imagining this state, you send a clear message to your subconscious mind, which in turn influences your physical reality. This practice can be enhanced by incorporating feelings of gratitude for your health as if it were already present. The combination of visualization and gratitude amplifies your intention, making it more likely to manifest in your life. Engaging in this practice regularly can lead to profound changes in your physical and emotional well-being.

Another vital aspect of the Law of Attraction in healing is the importance of surrounding ourselves with positive influences. The people, environments, and media we engage with can either uplift us or drain our energy. By consciously choosing to immerse ourselves in positivity—be it through supportive relationships, inspiring content, or nurturing spaces—we create a fertile ground for healing. This supportive atmosphere encourages us to maintain our focus on wellness and abundance, reinforcing the belief that we deserve to be healthy and happy. The synergy between our environment and our mindset becomes a powerful catalyst for transformation.

Finally, it is essential to remember that the Law of Attraction works in harmony with our actions. While positive thinking and visualization are vital components, they must be complemented by proactive steps towards health. This can include making healthier lifestyle choices, seeking medical advice when necessary, and engaging in activities that bring us joy and fulfillment. When we align our thoughts, emotions, and actions, we create a powerful trifecta that propels us toward healing. Embracing the Law of Attraction in our healing journey allows us to tap into our innate power, reminding us that we are co-creators of our health and happiness, capable of manifesting profound transformations in our lives.

Using Visualization and Journaling for Self-Healing

* * *

Visualization and journaling are powerful tools that can significantly enhance the self-healing journey. When we visualize, we engage our minds in a process that creates vivid images of our desires, aspirations, and healing outcomes. This practice taps into the subconscious, allowing us to overcome mental barriers and cultivate a positive mindset. Imagine picturing yourself free from pain, surrounded by light, or achieving your personal goals. Each image you create acts as a beacon, guiding your thoughts and actions toward that desired reality. The mind is incredibly potent, and by harnessing its power through visualization, we can effectively shift our emotional and physical states.

Journaling complements visualization beautifully by providing a space for reflection and expression. This practice allows us to articulate feelings, explore thoughts, and document our healing progress. Writing in a journal can be therapeutic; it helps in processing emotions that might otherwise remain bottled up. When we put pen to paper, we engage in a dialogue with ourselves, uncovering insights and realizations that are often hidden beneath the surface. By regularly journaling about our experiences, we create a tangible record of our journey, enabling us to track patterns, celebrate victories, and understand challenges more deeply.

Integrating visualization and journaling into a daily routine can amplify their effects, creating a synergistic approach to self-healing. Start your day with a brief visualization session, imagining your goals and the feelings associated with achieving them. Then, transition into journaling, capturing the essence of your visualization and any emotions that surface. This combination sets a positive tone for the day, reinforcing your intentions and providing clarity on your healing journey. The act of writing can serve as a grounding practice, solidifying your visualizations into actionable steps and affirmations you can carry with you.

Moreover, don't hesitate to get creative with these practices. Experiment with different visualization techniques, such as guided imagery or vision boards. In your journaling, you can weave in poetry, sketches, or even collages that resonate with your healing process. The key is to make these practices uniquely yours, allowing your personality and creativity to shine through. This personalized approach not only makes the process enjoyable but also deepens your connection to the work you're doing for yourself.

As you continue to explore visualization and journaling, remember that they are not just tools but gateways to self-discovery and empowerment. Embrace the journey, and allow these practices to guide you toward a greater understanding of yourself. Each session is an opportunity to release what no longer serves you, cultivate gratitude, and invite healing into your life. With consistency, patience, and an open heart, you will find that visualization and journaling can transform your experience of self-healing, revealing the extraordinary potential that lies within you.

Aligning Thoughts, Actions, and Energy for Ultimate Wellness

* * *

Aligning thoughts, actions, and energy is a transformative practice that lies at the heart of ultimate wellness. When these three elements are in harmony, they create a powerful synergy that supports self-healing and personal growth. Imagine your mind, body, and spirit working together seamlessly, like a well-tuned orchestra, producing a symphony of health and vitality. This alignment is not only essential for maintaining physical wellness but also for enhancing emotional resilience and spiritual depth. By consciously aligning these aspects of yourself, you unlock the door to profound healing experiences.

To begin this journey, start with your thoughts. Your mind is a powerful tool that can either uplift or undermine your wellness. Engage in practices such as mindfulness and positive affirmations to cultivate an optimistic mindset. Visualize your goals and dreams vividly, allowing them to fill your consciousness. When you focus on positive thoughts, you create a magnetic energy that attracts similar vibrations into your life. This mental clarity paves the way for intentional actions that resonate with your true self, rather than leading you astray into negativity or doubt.

Next, it's crucial to translate those thoughts into deliberate actions. Each decision you make is a reflection of your inner state, and when your actions align with your intentions, you create a pathway to wellness. Set achievable goals that resonate with your values and passions. Whether it's adopting healthier habits, engaging in creative pursuits, or nurturing relationships, ensure that every action you take is infused with purpose. This intentionality not only strengthens your self-discipline but also reinforces the positive thoughts you cultivate, creating a self-sustaining cycle of growth and well-being.

Energy is the final piece of this alignment puzzle. Your energy, both physical and emotional, plays a significant role in your overall wellness. Engage in practices that elevate your energy levels, such as yoga, meditation, or spending time in nature. These activities help you tap into your inner reservoir of vitality and connect with the universal life force. Pay attention to the energy you emit; it has the power to influence your surroundings and relationships. When you radiate positive energy, you create an environment that fosters healing, not just for yourself but also for those around you.

Ultimately, the journey of aligning thoughts, actions, and energy is a continuous process. Embrace it as a dynamic exploration rather than a fixed destination. Celebrate your progress, no matter how small, and remain open to the lessons that come your way. As you cultivate this alignment, you will find that ultimate wellness is not merely a state of being but a vibrant, evolving experience. Trust in your ability to heal, grow, and thrive, and watch as the universe responds to your newfound harmony with endless opportunities for joy and fulfillment.

CHAPTER 16: DESIGNING A MYSTIC HEALING LIFESTYLE

* * *

Daily Habits for Sustained Energy and Well-Being

Daily habits play a crucial role in maintaining sustained energy and well-being. By integrating simple yet powerful practices into your routine, you can unlock a vibrant life filled with vitality and joy. One of the most effective ways to start is by establishing a morning ritual that sets a positive tone for the day. Consider waking up a little earlier to engage in activities that nourish your spirit, such as meditation, journaling, or gentle stretching. These practices help ground you, allowing for clarity of mind and a boost in energy that carries you through your day.

Nutrition is another cornerstone of sustained energy and well-being. Choosing whole, nutrient-dense foods not only fuels your body but also supports your emotional and mental health. Incorporate a colorful variety of fruits and vegetables, whole grains, healthy fats, and lean proteins into your meals. The more diverse your diet, the more nutrients your body receives, leading to improved energy levels and overall well-being. Additionally, stay hydrated by drinking plenty of water throughout the day. This simple habit can significantly enhance your physical vitality and mental clarity.

Physical activity is essential for maintaining energy and promoting a sense of well-being. You don't need to engage in high-intensity workouts; even moderate exercise, such as walking, dancing, or yoga, can elevate your mood and increase your energy levels. Aim for at least 30 minutes of physical activity each day. This not only helps to release endorphins, the body's natural mood lifters, but also enhances your overall health, making you feel more alive and engaged with the world around you.

Mindfulness and self-care practices are equally important for fostering sustained energy. Taking time each day to check in with yourself, whether through meditation, deep breathing exercises, or simply sitting in silence, allows you to reconnect with your inner self. This helps to reduce stress and anxiety, which can drain your energy. Additionally, prioritize self-care activities that bring you joy, such as reading, spending time in nature, or indulging in a warm bath. These moments of self-nurturing recharge your spirit and cultivate a deeper sense of well-being.

Lastly, fostering positive relationships and connecting with others is vital for sustaining energy and well-being. Surround yourself with individuals who uplift and inspire you. Engage in meaningful conversations, share experiences, and participate in community activities that resonate with your values. Social connections not only enhance your emotional health but also provide support during challenging times. By prioritizing these daily habits, you can create a robust foundation for sustained energy and well-being, allowing you to thrive in every aspect of your life.

How to Integrate Mystic Healing into a Busy Modern Life

* * *

In the fast-paced world we live in today, finding time for self-care and healing can often feel like a daunting task. However, integrating mystic healing into your busy life is not only possible but can also be incredibly rewarding. The key lies in making small yet impactful changes to your daily routine. Start by carving out just a few moments each day dedicated to your well-being. This could be as simple as taking a mindful break during lunch or setting aside ten minutes in the morning for meditation. By treating these moments as sacred, you can begin to weave mystic healing into the fabric of your everyday life.

One effective approach is to incorporate elements of mystic healing into your existing activities. For instance, while you're commuting, turn your vehicle into a sanctuary of calm. Listen to guided meditations or soothing music that resonates with your spirit. Even if you're stuck in traffic, you can practice deep breathing techniques to center yourself. When you approach routine tasks like washing dishes or exercising, infuse them with intention. Visualize the cleansing of your spirit with each movement, transforming mundane chores into opportunities for healing and mindfulness.

Establishing a personal ritual can also elevate your experience of mystic healing. Whether it's lighting a candle while you sip your morning coffee or creating a nighttime gratitude practice, rituals serve as powerful anchors in your busy life. Choose a time that works for you—perhaps after a long day or at the start of a new one—and dedicate it to your ritual. This commitment to yourself can provide a sense of stability and remind you of the sacredness of your journey, even amidst the chaos of daily responsibilities.

Community is another vital element in integrating mystic healing into your life. Seek out local groups or online forums that align with your interests in mystic practices. Engaging with like-minded individuals can provide you with support, inspiration, and new ideas on how to incorporate healing into your routine. Whether it's a weekly yoga class, a book club focused on spiritual literature, or a meditation group, surrounding yourself with others on similar paths can reignite your enthusiasm and commitment to your own healing journey.

Finally, remember that integrating mystic healing into your life is a personal journey, and it's essential to approach it with compassion and flexibility. Life can be unpredictable, and there will be days when your routine gets interrupted. Embrace these moments and allow them to teach you about resilience and adaptability. Celebrate your progress, no matter how small, and understand that every effort you make contributes to your overall well-being. By nurturing this connection to mystic healing, you'll discover that it not only enriches your life but also empowers you to navigate the complexities of modern living with grace and clarity.

The Future of Self-Healing and Quantum Consciousness

* * *

The intersection of self-healing and quantum consciousness presents a thrilling frontier for exploration and transformation. As we dive deeper into the mysteries of our own existence, we begin to recognize that our thoughts, emotions, and intentions hold incredible power. This realization opens doors to profound healing possibilities, inviting us to harness the energy of our consciousness to not only heal ourselves but also to reshape our realities. Imagine a future where the principles of quantum physics intertwine with spiritual practices, creating a dynamic approach to health and well-being that transcends conventional boundaries.

In this new paradigm, self-healing becomes a vibrant dance between mind, body, and spirit. Quantum consciousness teaches us that we are not separate entities but rather interconnected beings vibrating within a vast web of energy. This understanding empowers us to tap into the infinite potential that lies within. As we embrace techniques that facilitate self-healing—such as meditation, visualization, and energy work—we begin to align ourselves with the quantum field, where healing is not just possible, but inevitable. The future of self-healing lies in our ability to consciously direct our energy towards wellness, making it an exhilarating journey of self-discovery.

The advancements in technology also play a pivotal role in shaping the future of self-healing and quantum consciousness. Innovations in biofeedback devices, wearable technology, and virtual reality experiences are providing us with unprecedented insights into our physiological and energetic states. These tools can amplify our self-healing practices, allowing us to monitor our progress and adjust our approaches in real-time. As we integrate these technologies into our healing journeys, we unlock new dimensions of awareness, creating a harmonious synergy between ancient wisdom and modern science.

Community and collective consciousness are equally vital in this evolving landscape. As we unite in our healing journeys, we amplify our intentions and elevate our collective vibration. Group meditations, healing circles, and online communities foster a sense of belonging and shared purpose. This interconnectedness not only enhances individual healing but also contributes to the greater good, as we collectively raise the consciousness of humanity. The future of self-healing is rooted in collaboration, where we support each other in our quests for wellness and enlightenment.

As we look ahead, the possibilities for self-healing and quantum consciousness are boundless. With each new discovery and practice, we step closer to realizing our innate potential. By embracing the principles of quantum mechanics and integrating them into our healing modalities, we can create a future where health and happiness are not just aspirations but realities. The journey is both personal and universal, inviting us to explore the depths of our being and the vastness of the universe. Together, we are pioneers on this thrilling path, unlocking the secrets of self-healing and quantum consciousness, and transforming our lives in ways we have yet to imagine.

MYSTIC
·WELLNESS LAB·

Unlocking the Science of Longevity, Energy & Healing

REVIEW REQUEST

DEAR READER

Thank you for reading Book. Your feedback is invaluable in helping others explore the insights within. If you found this book helpful or insightful, we kindly invite you to share a brief, honest review.

Warm regards,
Mystic Wellness Lab

www.ingramcontent.com/pod-product-compliance
Lightning Source LLC
La Vergne TN
LVHW090426210926
848480LV00002B/696
* 9 7 9 8 2 3 0 6 3 4 8 7 4 *